CME Registration Instructions

This Continuing Medical Education
project is sponsored by the
University of Virginia School of Medicine

Accreditation Statement

The University of Virginia School of Medicine is accredited by the Accreditation Council for Continuing Medical Education to provide continuing medical education for physicians.

The University of Virginia School of Medicine designates this educational activity for a maximum of 6.0 category 1 credits toward the AMA Physician's Recognition Award. Each physician should claim only those hours of credit that he or she actually spent in the educational activity.

The University of Virginia School of Medicine awards 0.1 Continuing Education Unit (CEU) per contact hour to each nonphysician participant who successfully completes this educational activity. The University of Virginia School of Medicine maintains a permanent record of participants who have been awarded CEUs.

The CME Quiz begins on page 305. Record your answers and fill out the information on the perforated Registration Form that is attached to the back cover. This information is required for a continuing medical education certificate. The Registration Form must be filled out completely for you to receive credit of 6.0 hours. Please print clearly. Mail the Registration Form to:

**University of Virginia Office of CME
Attn: Pam MacIntyre Box 800711
Charlottesville, VA 22908-0711**

Support for this activity was provided by an unrestricted educational grant from Pfizer Inc and Eisai

Disclosure of Faculty Financial Affiliations

As a provider accredited by the Accreditation Council for Continuing Medical Education, the Office of Continuing Medical Education of the University of Virginia School of Medicine must insure balance, independence, objectivity, and scientific rigor in all its individually sponsored or jointly sponsored educational activities. All faculty participating in a sponsored activity are expected to disclose to the activity audience any significant financial interest or other relationship. The intent of this disclosure is not to prevent a speaker with a significant financial or other reletionship from making a presentation, but rather to provide listeners with information on which they can make their own judgments. It remains for the audience to determine whether the speaker's interests or relationships may influence the presentation with regard to exposition or conclusion.

As required by the University of Virginia School of Medicine, David S. Geldmacher, MD, disclosed that he has received research support, consultant fees, and speaker's honoraria from Pfizer Inc and Eisai and research support from Janssen Pharmaceutica.

Elizabeth Crooks, RN, MSN, declared that she has no financial interest or other relationship with the manufacturer of any of the products or providers cited in this book.

Stephen J. Modafferi, Esq, declared that he has included discussion of commercial products and/or services but that he has no financial interest or other relationship with the manufacturer of any of the products or providers cited in this book.

Disclosure of Discussion of Non-FDA Approved Uses for Pharmaceutical Products and/or Medical Devices

The University of Virginia School of Medicine, as an ACCME provider, requires that all faculty presenters identify and disclose any off label uses for pharmaceutical and medical device products. The University of Virginia School of Medicine recommends that each physician fully review all the available data on new products or procedures before instituting them with patients. There is no discussion of non-FDA approved uses in this book.

Contemporary Diagnosis and Management of

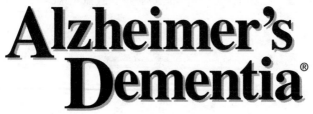

Alzheimer's Dementia®

David S. Geldmacher, MD

Associate Professor
Director, Memory Disorders Program
University of Virginia
Charlottesville, Virginia

First Edition

Published by Handbooks in Health Care Co.,
Newtown, Pennsylvania, USA

Dedication

This volume is dedicated to my parents, Joan E. Geldmacher and the late John F. Geldmacher, who laid the foundations for any successes I may achieve.

International Standard Book Number: 1-931981-16-7

Library of Congress Catalog Card Number: 2003104636

Table of Contents

This book has been prepared and is presented as a service to the medical community. The information provided reflects the knowledge, experience, and personal opinions of the author, David S. Geldmacher, MD, Associate Professor, Director, Memory Disorders Program, University of Virginia, Charlottesville, Virginia.

Chapter 1

Introduction: History, Epidemiology, and Public Health Issues

Alzheimer's disease (AD) is now recognized as the most common cause of late-life dementia worldwide. It is poised to become an overwhelming public health issue in developed nations during the first half of the 21st century. AD may pose an even greater threat to social structure in immense developing nations like China and India, where the aging of the population lags behind Europe and North America. AD is considered the third most expensive illness in the United States, with a total economic burden already estimated at $60 billion to $100 billion annually. These costs are even more ominous when considering that the prevalence of AD in the United States has been projected to grow from between 4 million and 5 million affected individuals in 2000 to nearly 15 million by 2050. These are astounding figures for an illness that had not yet been recognized at the outset of the 20th century.

History

In 1901, the German neurologist Dr. Alois Alzheimer examined a 51-year-old woman from Frankfurt (Figure 1). Her name was Auguste, and she had a 4-year history of delusional jealousy and progressive cognitive decline. The cause of her illness was not known, and he followed her until her death 5 years later. During that time, Dr. Alzhei-

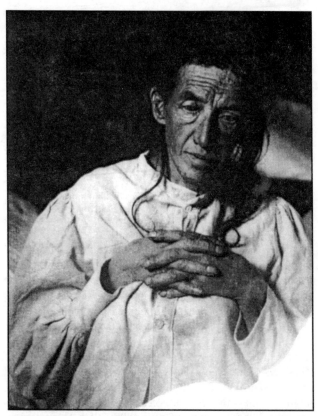

Figure 1: Photograph of Auguste, circa 1904. She was the first person ever recognized to have the illness now called Alzheimer's disease.

mer recorded her progressive disability from cognitive impairments. (A fascinating review of his original case notes was published by Maurer et al in 1997.[1]) Auguste developed difficulties with language, skilled movement (praxis), and decision making. After her death in 1906, Alzheimer and his laboratory team performed a neuropathologic examination of her brain, using recently developed staining techniques. Alzheimer reported their results in 1906 and 1907 in German as a "strange ailment of the cerebral cortex."[2] The principal findings were the pathologic structures now called senile plaques and neurofibrillary tangles, which remain mandatory neuropathologic features for this syndrome even today. Kraepelin was the first to refer to this 'strange ailment' as *Alzheimer's disease* in his text several years later.

Nomenclature

Although it was not routinely called so during her life, Auguste had dementia. Dementia comes from the Latin *de mens*, literally 'out of the mind.' In colloquial use, it is often equated with primary mental illness (ie, demented = crazy). In health care, however, dementia is defined as impaired memory with a loss of other cognitive abilities or change in personality sufficiently severe to interfere with previously achieved levels of daily function.[3] The word *dementia* itself describes a clinical state, and implies neither cause nor course. However, dementia is commonly used to describe the underlying brain disease, as well as its clinical manifestation. The more accurate, though often cumbersome, terminology differentiates the clinical state of dementia from the causative dementing illness, eg, dementia of the Alzheimer type vs Alzheimer's disease. This differentiation becomes especially important when planning treatment approaches that might ameliorate the symptoms but not affect the course. Similarly, treatments might be instituted that alter disease progression but do not improve symptoms acutely. In Alzheimer's disease, both strategies can be used (see Chapters 7, 8, and 9).

Cognitive decline has been associated with late life since antiquity. Its frequency is perhaps best identified in the historic use of the word *senility* as a synonym for the loss of cognitive abilities in old age. Senility, however, means only the state of being old. Alzheimer's case proved that old age was not a requirement for a decline in cognitive function in an otherwise physically healthy and mentally intact person. Nonetheless, for more than 50 years, AD was considered an odd and unusual form of early-onset (presenile) dementia that was somehow different from what happened to older adults. In the mid-1960s, the British group of Blessed, Tomlinson, and Roth[4] fundamentally influenced the medical and scientific approach to dementia when they published the finding that the plaques and tangles of AD were strongly associated with cognitive loss in older adults. Subsequently, the knowledge of AD has grown exponentially, and a revolution is underway in thinking about the aging brain and its illnesses.

Other synonyms for dementia that have been superseded include *cerebral atherosclerosis* and its lay equivalent, *hardening of the arteries*. These terms were based on the mistaken impression that cognitive impairment was caused by a chronic state of oxygen starvation in the brain resulting from tissue hypoperfusion. Although cerebral infarcts can indeed cause dementia, there is little evidence for chronic ischemia without infarction or other forms of irreversible damage. Another obsolete term for dementia is *organic brain syndrome*. This term has some historical importance because it acknowledged that the behavioral and cognitive symptoms of dementia have a neurologic (organic) rather than psychiatric origin. Nonetheless, the phrase lacks any etymologic meaning, since it can be translated as 'a brain syndrome arising from the brain.' It thus also fails to convey any pathophysiologic or clinical specificity. Therefore, although this diagnosis persists in the International Classification of Diseases (ICD), it should not be used.

Epidemiology

AD is the most common cause of dementia in nearly all populations studied. In most reports, AD accounts for about two thirds of new cases of dementia in people over age 65. The incidence rates reported for dementia (ie, the number of new cases evolving in a population over a set interval) vary widely. Methodologic differences and variability in diagnostic schema account for more of the variation between reports than intrinsic differences in the populations under study. Age is the chief risk factor for the development of AD, and it must be considered vital to any estimate of incidence. Despite its original recognition as a presenile dementia, AD occurring before age 65 is rare. Incidence rates for people 40 to 64 years old have been estimated between 0.2 and 0.4 new cases per 1,000 population per year. From ages 65 to 69, the estimated incidence of AD ranges from about 0.7 to 3.5 per 1,000 annually, and doubles approximately every 5 years.[5] By age 90, the incidence may be more than 65 per 1,000 per year. The overwhelming nature of this disease frequency is expressed by Aevarsson and Skoog, who reported in 1996 that between ages 85 and 88, almost 10% of nondemented persons become demented each year.[6]

Prevalence refers to the number of cases in a population at a given time. As with incidence, estimates vary widely. Broad measures of dementia prevalence in developed countries suggest an overall rate between 4% and 8% over age 65, but these figures do not account for mild cases that have not come to medical attention or formal diagnosis. One useful model is to consider the prevalence of AD at age 60 to be about 1%, and to assume that the rate will double every 5 years, leading to predicted prevalences of 2% at age 65, 4% at 70, 8% at 75, 16% at 80, and 30%+ by age 85.[7] Because of comorbidities and reduced life expectancy from all causes, the rate of increase in the prevalence of AD may slow slightly after age 85. Nonetheless, prevalence rates of 40% in people aged 90 to 94, and 58% in those 95 and above, have been reported.[8]

Major Risk Factors

Family history is an exceptionally potent risk factor for AD, second only in importance to age. Several mu-

Table 1: Risk Factors for Alzheimer's Disease

Established

- Age
- Specific mutations on chromosomes 1, 14, and 21
- Family history of dementia
- Down syndrome
- Apolipoprotein E ε-4 genotype

Possible*

- Low education
- Female gender
- Depression
- Brain injury

* Many others have been reported, but evidence is weak, preliminary, or controversial.

tations are associated with autosomal-dominant early-onset familial AD. These are characterized by expression of AD in sequential generations, usually with onset during the fifth or sixth decade. Mutations have been identified on chromosomes 1, 14, and 21 in these kindreds. Commercial and academic laboratory testing for these genetic anomalies is available for individuals in these kindreds, and may be valuable in genetic counseling and health-care planning, such as for advance directives and insurance purchases. It is important to recognize, however, that these genetic loci account for only a minority of cases of early-onset familial AD, and therefore for a very small proportion of the overall population with AD (Table 1).

Down syndrome (DS), or the clinical manifestation of trisomy 21, is another clearly identified risk factor. Nearly 100% of individuals with DS develop the neuropathologic changes of AD by the sixth decade. Clinical evidence for dementia may be hard to detect because of the incomplete intellectual development in DS, but newly evolving behavioral symptoms during adulthood warrant consideration of AD as a contributor. The very high risk for AD in Down syndrome is likely associated with overproduction of the amyloid precursor protein (APP), the gene for which is located on chromosome 21. The mechanisms that lead to AD in Down syndrome are therefore likely to be similar to the pathophysiologic process among kindreds with autosomal-dominant chromosome 21 mutations. A family history of DS may also convey a slightly increased risk for AD, because translocation or chromosomal nondisjunction events can lead to duplication of the APP gene without the full trisomy syndrome.

Even in the absence of an autosomal-dominant inheritance pattern or DS, family history conveys significant risk. Data from the Multi-Institutional Research in Alzheimer Genetic Epidemiology (MIRAGE) project suggest that individuals with an affected first-degree relative show about a 40% cumulative lifetime risk of developing AD. Those with 2 affected parents had a 54% risk of developing AD by age 80, but the impact of family history appears reduced after age 90.[9] A family history of dementia-free longevity has the reverse effect. The risk of dementia in relatives of people reaching old age without dementia is one third the risk for randomly selected individuals, and one tenth the risk for relatives of AD patients.[10]

Apolipoprotein E genotype contributes to the effect of family history on overall risk. Apolipoprotein E (ApoE) is a lipid-carrying plasma protein encoded on chromosome 19. It is expressed in three allelic forms, epsilon-2, -3, and -4 (ϵ-2, ϵ-3, and ϵ-4). Many studies have shown that the ϵ-4 allele is associated with an increased risk for developing AD,

Table 2: Possible Protective Factors*
Against Alzheimer's Disease

- Dementia-free family history

- Apolipoprotein E ε-2 genotype

- High education or socioeconomic status

- Chronic nonsteroidal anti-inflammatory drug therapy

* Many others have been reported, but evidence is weak, preliminary, or controversial.

particularly late-onset familial disease. There appears to be a dose effect as well, with ε-4 homozygotes developing AD at earlier ages than heterozygotes. Homozygosity for ε-4 was associated with a 30-fold increase in AD risk in one study, which also showed a nearly 4-fold increased risk for ε-3/ε-4 heterozygotes.[11] The ε-3 allele is most frequent in most populations and appears to be neutral in its risk for development of AD. The rare ε-2 allele may convey a slight protective effect (Table 2), since AD is absent among ε-2 carriers in some studies, even if ε-4 is also present.[11] Interestingly, the strong risk effect of ε-4 in European and North American populations may not be equivalent in other populations.[12]

Also, method of study strongly affects the relative impact of ApoE status on AD risk. Prospective population studies tend to show less of an ApoE effect than do autopsy-based series. Despite a clear role as a risk factor, it is important to note that ε-4 is not required for the development of AD, because ε-4-negative individuals account for about 50% of AD cases.[11] One estimate of its impact suggests that if ε-4 did not exist or was risk-neutral, AD incidence would be reduced by only 13.7%.[13] Like age and family history, ApoE genotype is an unmodifiable risk factor.

Putative Risk Factors

Although the evidence is not as clear as for previously discussed factors, some risk factors for AD may be subject to manipulation (Table 1). Individuals with low education or low lifetime achievements have been reported to develop AD at more than twice the rate than those with more education and achievement.[14] A study conducted in East Boston, Massachusetts suggested that the risk for developing AD was reduced by 17% for each year of education.[15] Prevalence rates are similarly reduced with increased education. A study of a rural Italian population found that persons with very low education (eg, less than 3 years) were twice as likely to have AD.[16] It is unclear how education and similar measures reduce AD risk, but practical considerations, such as greater experience with test situations, must be considered as much as more theoretical models, such as increased synaptic density or enhanced cognitive reserve.

Depression may also be an increased risk factor for dementia. Devanand et al reported in 1996 that depressed individuals over age 60 had a 2-to-4 times increased risk of developing AD over a 5-year follow-up period.[17] Whether the depression represents an early sign of AD or increases susceptibility to the illness through other mechanisms is unknown. Past head injury is another factor that may contribute to increased risk or earlier onset.[18] An intriguing interaction of ApoE ε-4 and history of head injury as combined risk factors for AD has also been reported.[19]

Female gender has been identified as a risk factor for AD in some studies, but not in others. The prevalence of dementia is clearly higher in women because more women than men live into the age range at risk. However, this effect sometimes disappears when data are controlled for age and differential survival. Some evidence indicates that postmenopausal estrogen replacement therapy may reduce AD risk.[20] Estrogens are also known to interact with trophic influences such as nerve growth factor, which suggests that the relative estrogen deprivation experienced by postmenopausal women may be a factor in their increased risk. Much further study will be required to clarify these complex relationships.

Similarly, chronic exposure to nonsteroidal anti-inflammatory drugs (NSAIDs) may convey a protective effect.[21] The frequency and severity of morbidity associated with long-term NSAID use, however, warrants significant caution in interpreting their overall risk and benefit to individuals at risk for AD. Neither estrogens nor NSAIDs are approved in the United States for use in prevention or treatment of AD. (For more discussion of potential disease-altering therapies, see Chapter 7.) Aluminum has been repeatedly implicated as a potential risk factor for AD. In fact, one form of dementia is strongly associated with aluminum content in renal dialysis fluids, but the evidence for a significant role of aluminum in the pathogenesis of AD is unconvincing.

Health Economics

The total economic burden of AD in the United States is estimated to be $100 billion annually, making it the third most expensive illness, following only heart disease and cancer.[22] Costs are generally less earlier in the illness, and increase with progression into more severe stages. The costs associated with AD have direct and indirect components. Direct costs include expenditures for nursing home care, in-home health assistance, outpatient day-care services, and medication. These represent 20% to 25% of total cost. Indirect costs include lost patient and caregiver productivity, including unreimbursed time spent in caregiving. Estimates from 1991 placed the annual cost of care at $47,581 per patient per year.[23] The same authors reported a total cost of more than $173,000 per Alzheimer's patient. These estimates suggest little difference in total annual cost between institutionalized AD patients and those who live at home with similar degrees of disease severity. However, the distribution of cost does differ with the site of care. The direct costs for institutionalized patients are 3 times higher. The shifting of care to paid workers concomitantly reduces the indirect costs sustained by families. Total economic burden, therefore, remains relatively independent of site of care.

Families pay about 60% of direct AD-related costs out of pocket.[24] About 75% of AD patients eventually require nursing home care and, once admitted, their length of stay is 10 times the national average for all diagnoses.[25] Institutional care requires payment of these direct costs in concrete forms (ie, cash). Medicare and most other health insurance plans cover almost no long-term care costs in nursing homes or similar facilities, so the *perceived* financial burden increases with placement in a long-term care setting.

The oldest of the old, with AD prevalence rates exceeding 30%, will constitute an increasing proportion of the US population through at least 2050, further magnifying the public health burden of this illness. Not all authorities support catastrophic economic projections based on current AD figures. Caution is indeed warranted in interpreting the projected costs, because if AD does not cause functional decline or death in these patients, some other illness will. Eliminating AD, therefore, might only shift the economic burden to other illnesses, making any cost savings illusory.

Another aspect of the public health burden associated with dementia is quality of life. Treatments that reduce costs but adversely affect the quality of life of persons with AD or their families may be economically feasible, but be at odds with the health care system's moral obligation to reduce suffering. Unfortunately, the questions of how to accurately and effectively measure quality of life in dementia, as well as weigh its impact, remain unanswered.

Conclusion

For the foreseeable future, individuals will continue to develop dementia from AD and other illnesses. Skilled clinicians will be needed to treat these devastating illnesses and lessen their impact on patients and families. The purpose of this book is to present the information necessary to diagnose dementia, differentiate between the illnesses that can lead to it, treat its symptoms appropriately, and favorably alter its course.

References

1. Maurer K, Volk S, Gerbaldo H: Auguste D and Alzheimer's disease. *Lancet* 1997;349:1546-1549.

2. Alzheimer A: Uber eine eigenartige erkangkung der hirnrinde. Allgemaine Zeitschrift fur Psychiatrie und Psychisch-Gerichtliche Medizin 1907;64:146-148. (English translation in: *Arch Neurol* 1967;21:109-110.)

3. American Psychiatric Association: *Diagnostic and Statistical Manual of Mental Disorders* (DSM-III-R), 3rd ed, revised. Washington, DC, 1987.

4. Blessed G, Tomlinson BE, Roth M: The association between quantitative measures of dementia and of senile change in the cerebral grey matter of elderly subjects. *Br J Psychiatry* 1968;114:797-811.

5. Bachman DL, Wolf PA, Linn RT, et al: Incidence of dementia and probable Alzheimer's disease in a general population: the Framingham Study. *Neurology* 1993;43:515-519.

6. Aevarsson O, Skoog I: A population-based study on the incidence of dementia disorders between 85 and 88 years of age. *J Am Geriatr Soc* 1996;44:1455-1460.

7. White LR, Cartwright WS, Cornoni-Huntley J, et al: Geriatric epidemiology. *Annu Rev Gerontol Geriatr* 1986;6:215-311.

8. Ebly EM, Parhad IM, Hogan DB, et al: Prevalence and types of dementia in the very old: results from the Canadian Study of Health and Aging. *Neurology* 1994;44:1593-1600.

9. Lautenschlager NT, Cupples LA, Rao VS, et al: Risk of dementia among relatives of Alzheimer's disease patients in the MIRAGE study: what is in store for the oldest old? *Neurology* 1996;46:641-650.

10. Payami H, Montee K, Kaye J: Evidence for familial factors that protect against dementia and outweigh the effect of increasing age. *Am J Hum Genet* 1994;54:650-657.

11. Myers RH, Schaefer EJ, Wilson PW, et al: Apolipoprotein E ε-4 association with dementia in a population-based study: the Framingham study. *Neurology* 1996;46:673-677.

12. Kalaria RN, Ogeng'o JA, Patel NB, et al: Evaluation of risk factors for Alzheimer's disease in elderly east Africans. *Brain Res Bull* 1997;44:573-577.

13. Evans DA, Beckett LA, Field TS, et al: Apolipoprotein E ε-4 and incidence of Alzheimer disease in a community population of older persons. *JAMA* 1997;277:822-824.

14. Stern Y, Gurland B, Tatemichi TK, et al: Influence of education and occupation on the incidence of Alzheimer's disease. *JAMA* 1994;271:1004-1010.

15. Evans DA, Hebert LE, Beckett LA, et al: Education and other measures of socioeconomic status and risk of incident Alzheimer disease in a defined population of older persons. *Arch Neurol* 1997;54:1399-1405.

16. Prencipe M, Casini AR, Ferretti C, et al: Prevalence of dementia in an elderly rural population: effects of age, sex, and education. *J Neurol Neurosurg Psychiatry* 1996;60:628-633.

17. Devanand DP, Sano M, Tang MX, et al: Depressed mood and the incidence of Alzheimer's disease in the elderly living in the community. *Arch Gen Psychiatry* 1996;53:175-182.

18. Schofield PW, Tang M, Marder K, et al: Alzheimer's disease after remote head injury: an incidence study. *J Neurol Neurosurg Psychiatry* 1997;62:119-124.

19. Mayeux R, Ottman R, Maestre G, et al: Synergistic effects of traumatic head injury and apolipoprotein-epsilon 4 in patients with Alzheimer's disease. *Neurology* 1995;45:555-557.

20. Tang MX, Jacobs D, Stern Y, et al: Effect of oestrogen during menopause on risk and age at onset of Alzheimer's disease. *Lancet* 1996;348:429-432.

21. McGeer PL, Schulzer M, McGeer EG: Arthritis and anti-inflammatory agents as possible protective factors for Alzheimer's disease: a review of 17 epidemiologic studies. *Neurology* 1996;47:425-432.

22. Meek PD, McKeithan K, Schumock GT: Economic considerations in Alzheimer's disease. *Pharmacotherapy* 1998;18:68-73.

23. Ernst RL, Hay JW: The US economic and social costs of Alzheimer's disease revisited. *Am J Public Health* 1994;84:1261-1264.

24. Rice DP, Fox PJ, Max W, et al: The economic burden of Alzheimer's disease care. *Health Aff (Millwood)* 1993;12:164-176.

Chapter 2

Basic Disease Mechanisms in AD

T he primary cause of AD remains unknown. None-theless, an explosive growth in knowledge has oc-curred regarding senile plaques and neurofibrillary tangles, which remain the primary pathologic markers of the illness nearly 100 years after their initial discovery. There have also been important breakthroughs in understanding the molecular genetics of AD. Consequently, a brief review of the neurobiologic underpinnings of basic disease mechanisms is necessary to more fully understand the clinical expression of AD.

Neuropathologic Findings

On gross examination at autopsy, the AD brain is usually atrophic with enlarged ventricles and sulci. Total brain weight is invariably reduced, but there is still significant overlap with the range of brain weights for normal older adults.

Senile Plaques

Senile plaques are one of the classic findings reported by Alzheimer. They are accumulations of amyloid, an abnormal proteinaceous material, and cellular elements. They range in diameter from 15μ to 100μ and are distributed throughout the gray matter of cortex and limbic nuclei. The highest concentrations are typically found in the hippocampus. Senile plaques take 2 major forms. *Neuritic plaques* have a high proportion of distorted presynaptic neuronal elements, known as neurites. These include paired helical filaments, lysosomes, and mitochondria. Microglia are typically found in and around a dense core of extracellular amyloid, while fibrillary astrocytes may be seen at the periphery. Other plaques that lack dense cores of amyloid peptide and large numbers of neurites are known as *diffuse plaques* and are not clearly associated with neuronal loss and cognitive dysfunction. Diffuse plaques, unlike neuritic plaques, are found in the cerebellum and spinal cord. Amyloid can also accumulate in cerebral blood vessels, a condition known as cerebral amyloid angiopathy. This leads to an increased risk for intracerebral lobar hemorrhage.

The form of amyloid deposited in the brains of patients with AD is known as beta-amyloid (Aβ), and is sometimes referred to as A4 or βA4. Aβ is a ~4kD peptide that consists of 39-43 amino acid fragments proteolytically derived from a family of transmembrane proteins, collectively known as β-amyloid precursor protein (βAPP). The differing forms of βAPP are encoded from a single gene located on the long arm of chromosome 21. βAPP's normal function is unknown, but it closely resembles a class of protease inhibitors, which includes the nexins and the inhibitor of clotting factor XIa. Normally, βAPP is enzymatically cleaved by α-secretase to release a long soluble N-terminal fragment into extracellular space. The residual C-terminal fragment is cleaved by γ-secretase, then internalized and degraded intracellularly. Presenilin-1 appears to be associated with β-secretase activity.

In AD, it appears that an increased proportion of βAPP is processed by β-secretases to leave the Aβ sequence intact. This results in the extracellular deposition of aggregates of Aβ in an insoluble β-pleated sheet configuration. Mutations in and around the βAPP sequence are associated with increased production of Aβ peptides that are usually 40, 42, or 43 amino acids in length. Deposition of the longer 42 or 43 amino acid residues of Aβ appears to be a fundamental pathophysiologic process in plaque development.

Neurons are the primary source of Aβ in the AD brain, but markers of Aβ activity are also found to be associated with astrocytes, microglia, and perivascular cells.

How Aβ contributes to neuronal dysfunction and death in AD is unknown. Glycoproteins similar to βAPP are associated with cell surface interactions and nuclear signaling, which suggests that βAPP or its normal derivatives might play a role in maintaining synaptic and neuronal health. Two-way communication across synaptic junctions is important for maintaining their viability. One hypothesis regarding the role of amyloid in triggering neuronal loss in AD involves disruption of the cytoskeleton of presynaptic neurons because of βAPP- or Aβ-induced synaptic disconnection.[1] Another possibility is that insoluble Aβ provokes an inflammatory reaction with neurotoxic side effects. In this model of AD, microglial cells react to the Aβ deposits, triggering an inflammatory cascade that ultimately leads to neuronal death. This cellular reaction distinguishes neuritic plaques associated with the disruption of neuronal architecture and function from the more benign diffuse amyloid plaques. The hypotheses about inflammation as a contributing factor to the progression of AD are well-supported, and have led to wider therapeutic possibilities than previously envisioned.[2-4]

Neurofibrillary Tangles

Neurofibrillary tangles (NFT) are the second classical finding in AD. NFTs are intracellular collections of abnormal filaments, which have a distinctive paired helical structure in AD. Other degenerative illnesses, such as progressive supranuclear palsy and dementia pugilistica, are characterized by NFTs that do not have the paired helical structure. NFTs are found throughout the neocortex and limbic nuclei, where they are closely correlated to the degree of cell loss. They are also strongly represented in the basal forebrain, substantia nigra, raphe nuclei, and locus ceruleus. NFTs only occasionally appear in the brains of nondemented older adults. In AD, NFTs occupy large areas within the cell bodies of affected pyramidal neurons. This class of neurons is responsible for long axonal projections that facilitate inter- and intrahemispheric communication. The components of NFTs include a protein known as *tau*, which binds to microtubules and maintains them in the polymerized state required for their normal function. Abnormal hyperphosphorylation of tau may interfere with its ability to stabilize intraneuronal microtubule arrays. Loss of tau's stabilizing effect leads microtubules to collapse and spontaneously aggregate into AD's characteristic paired helical filaments.[5] After cell death, 'ghost tangles' remain in the extracellular matrix and mark the sites of dead neurons.

Neuropil threads (NT) are another neuropathologic finding in AD that is related to NFT. NTs are found scattered in the cerebral cortical extracellular matrix. Like NFTs, they consist of paired helical filamentous structures, and are also found clustered among the dystrophic neurites of senile plaques.

Synaptic Loss

Widespread cortical synaptic loss occurs in AD and is perhaps the major determinant of cognitive disability in the disease. The deep layers of the temporal cortex and the hippocampus appear most affected. In addition, synaptic inputs to the cortex are reduced up to 40% by the time of death.[6] Synaptic communication is the essence of forebrain function, so it is not surprising that the degree of synapse loss in the frontal cortex correlates well with cognitive impairment in AD.[7] Loss of frontal synaptic inputs is closely tied to dysfunction in the parietal lobe association cortex, which is a primary site for NFT and loss of pyramidal neurons responsible for long intrahemispheric axonal connections.

Substantial neuronal dropout also occurs in the basal forebrain nuclei, such as the nucleus basalis of Meynert, which produce the neurotransmitter acetylcholine. The number of NFTs in these deep forebrain cholinergic nuclei closely relates to the degree of memory loss in AD.[6] Synapses and cells are lost in the locus ceruleus and the raphe nuclei. Neurons in these brainstem nuclei produce monoamine neurotransmitters and distribute them in the cerebral cortex via long ascending axons.

Other Microscopic Findings

Granulovacuolar degeneration is common in AD, but is also known to occur to a lesser degree in normal aging. In demented patients, the pyramidal cell areas of the hippocampus seem to be particularly prone to the development of these 5μ-diameter, clear, intracytoplasmic vacuoles with argyrophilic cores. Several vacuoles can be seen in some neurons. Hirano bodies are eosinophilic cellular inclusions that are also in the hippocampal pyramidal layer. They are composed primarily of crystalline arrays of actin. Like the granulovacuolar changes, Hirano bodies can be seen in healthy aging, but in markedly lower numbers than seen in AD.

Neurochemical Findings

The primary function of neurons is communication with other neurons. Interneuronal communication is accomplished by release and reception of neurotransmitters at the synapse. Neurotransmitter changes are therefore an important part of the functional changes in AD.

Acetylcholine

A correlation exists between the severity of Alzheimer's dementia and loss of cerebral cortical markers for acetylcholine (ACh) metabolism. These markers include the synthetic enzyme choline acetyltransferase (CAT) and the degradative enzyme acetylcholinesterase (AChE). The degree of cholinergic reduction in the cortex is closely associated with the amount of cellular loss in the basal forebrain nuclei, where the neurons that produce much of the cortical ACh are located.[8]

Table 1: Genetic Features of Early-Onset Familial AD

Location	Gene Product	Proportion of Early-Onset AD
Chromosome 1	Presenilin-2	<1%
Chromosome 14	Presenilin-1	18% to 50%
Chromosome 21	β-Amyloid Precursor Protein	<5%

Also, AChE receptor changes occur in AD. Several subtypes of cholinergic receptors have been identified. These include the muscarinic receptors located on postsynaptic intracortical cells (known as M1 receptors) and the presynaptic M2 receptors located near the nerve terminals of ascending cholinergic axons. Generally, the M1 receptors are preserved in AD but the M2 sites are markedly reduced.[9] Nicotinic cholinergic receptors are probably also presynaptic, but unlike the M2 sites, they are likely to promote the release of ACh. Acetylcholine is important in the cognitive functions of attention and memory. The possibility that these symptoms might improve with cholinergic augmentation accounts for much of the emphasis on developing further understanding of cholinergic dysfunction in AD. Potential drug therapies could be designed to strengthen cholinergic function by enhancing production via CAT, decreasing degradation by AChE, stimulating M1 or nicotinic receptors, or inhibiting M2 receptors.

Monoamines

The cognitive and behavioral disturbances of AD do not result simply from cholinergic deficits. Other ascending pathways, such as those for norepinephrine (NE) and serotonin (5-HT), are also affected and may contribute to both cognitive and noncognitive symptoms. NE is important for arousal, learning, and memory. The major site for NE production is the locus ceruleus in the brainstem, which undergoes significant cell loss in AD.[10] AD is also associated with decreased markers of 5-HT activity in the cortex and loss of 5-HT-producing cells in the raphe nuclei of the brainstem.[10] Changes in the monoamine transmitters NE and 5-HT are likely to contribute to mood, anxiety, and other behavioral disturbances in AD patients.[10,11] Intrinsic classical neurotransmitters, such as gamma-aminobutyric acid (GABA), are also diminished, as are many cortically localized neuropeptides, such as somatostatin and corticotropin releasing factor. The role of these changes in the AD clinical syndrome is unknown.

Genetic Factors

Familial forms of AD were first recognized in the 1920s. We now recognize several types of autosomal dominant familial AD with nearly complete penetrance. These cases almost always begin before age 60 and are linked to known mutations on chromosomes 21, 14, and 1.[12] It is important to recognize that less than half of early-onset AD cases are associated with these mutations (Table 1). The known genetic causes, therefore, account for only about 5% of all AD. Screening for candidate genes is a rapidly growing area of research in AD, but the results can be confusing.[13,14]

Genetic epidemiology also suggests that AD should not be considered a purely genetic disease. Twin studies, for example, suggest a concordance of only 40% to 50% in monozygotic twin pairs. Nonetheless, much of the current understanding of the molecular biologic bases of AD has arisen from study of familial cases.

Chromosome 21

The first clues to the molecular biologic basis of AD came from families with an autosomal dominant pattern of inheritance that was linked to the βAPP region on the long arm of chromosome 21. There are several kindreds with different mutations in the βAPP sequence. These families account for less than 5% of all early-onset familial AD and less than 0.5% of all AD cases. The mutations are presumed to interfere with the normal proteolytic processing of βAPP and lead to deposition of insoluble Aβ. Another chromosome 21-related form of AD is found in individuals with Down syndrome or trisomy 21. Instead of a mutated gene, these individuals (and sometimes family members) receive 3 copies of βAPP. The extra βAPP may overwhelm the normal α-secretase proteolytic pathway, leading to increased Aβ formation, deposition, and neurotoxicity.

Chromosome 14

A significantly more common source for early-onset familial AD is localized to chromosome 14. Dozens of point mutations have been found in a region encoding the 467-amino acid protein now known as presenilin 1 (PS-1). The PS-1 gene is homologous to genes found in *Drosophila* flies and in primitive organisms like *Caenorhabditis elegans*, suggesting a highly conserved function for the PS-1 protein. The function of that protein is unknown, but its structure includes 6 apparent transmembrane segments. PS-1 mutations account for 18% to 50% of all early-onset familial AD. Commercial testing for PS-1 mutations is available, but it should only be obtained in families with early-onset AD and only when accompanied by thorough genetic counseling to assist with the interpretation of the results and their implications.

Chromosome 1

After the discovery of the PS-1 gene, a nucleotide sequence was subsequently identified on chromosome 1 that has a high degree of homology with PS-1. This region encodes a 447-amino acid protein that is 67% homologous with PS-1 and is now known as PS-2. The chromosome 1 region for PS-2 is linked with early-onset AD in a group of Volga German families. The mutations associated with PS-2 are in the second transmembrane domain of the protein, an area that is the site of many of the PS-1 mutations. Mutations in this gene are a very rare cause of early-onset familial AD.

Conclusion

Despite rapidly increasing knowledge about the pathophysiologic mechanisms associated with AD, there is no consensus about how the process begins. The fact that very different genetic lesions lead to identical clinical and pathologic outcomes means that a complex multifactorial process must be involved. The neurobiologic understanding of AD is further complicated by relatively low concordance in twin studies, the frequency of nonfamilial cases, and the lack of any clear environmental links. From the clinician's perspective, the most promising lines of investigation for the immediate future are those associated with the role of inflammation in triggering or propagating the cascade of events that result in cellular and synaptic loss in AD. These studies are most likely to uncover the next generation of disease-altering therapies. Pharmaceuticals or genetic techniques to prevent or minimize the deposition of insoluble Aβ remain a viable long-term goal of the research approaches to AD.

References

1.   Sisodia SS, Price DL: Amyloidogenesis in Alzheimer's disease. *Clin Neurosci* 1993;1:176-183.

2.   Breitner JC: Inflammatory processes and antiinflammatory drugs in Alzheimer's disease: a current appraisal. *Neurobiol Aging* 1996;17:789-794.

3.   Kalaria RN, Cohen DL, Premkumar DR: Cellular aspects of the inflammatory response in Alzheimer's disease. *Neurodegeneration* 1996;5:497-503.

4.   Aisen PS: Inflammation and Alzheimer's disease: mechanisms and therapeutic strategies. *Gerontology* 1997;43:143-149.

5.   Goedert M: Tau protein and the neurofibrillary pathology of Alzheimer's disease. *Ann NY Acad Sci* 1996;777:121-131.

6.   Masliah E, Terry RD: Role of synaptic pathology in the mechanisms of dementia of the Alzheimer's type. *Clin Neurosci* 1993;1:192-198.

7.   Dekosky ST, Scheff SW: Synapse loss in frontal cortex biopsies in Alzheimer's disease: correlation with cognitive severity. *Ann Neurol* 1990;27:457-464.

8.   Whitehouse PJ, Price DL, Clark AW, et al: Alzheimer's disease: evidence for selective loss of cholinergic neurons in the nucleus basalis. *Ann Neurol* 1981;10:122-126.

9.   Ladinsky HL, Schiavi GB, Honferini E, et al: Pharmacological muscarinic receptor subtypes. *Prog Brain Res* 1990;84:193-200.

10.   Zweig RM, Ross CA, Hedreen JC, et al: The neuropathology of aminergic nuclei in Alzheimer's disease. *Ann Neurol* 1988;24:233-242.

11.   Zubenko GS, Moosy J, Martinez AJ, et al: Neuropathologic and neurochemical correlates of psychosis in primary dementia. *Ann Neurol* 1991;48:619-624.

12.   Levy-Lahad E, Tsuang D, Bird TD: Recent advances in the genetics of Alzheimer's disease. *J Geriatr Psychiatry Neurol* 1998;11:42-54.

13.   Rogaeva E, Premkumar S, Song Y, et al: Evidence for an Alzheimer disease susceptibility locus on chromosome 12 and for further further locus heterogeneity. *JAMA* 1998;280:614-618.

14.   Wu WS, Holmans P, Wavrant-DeVrieze F, et al: Genetic studies on chromosome 12 in late-onset Alzheimer disease. *JAMA* 1998;280:619-622.

Chapter 3

Clinical Expression of AD

T he primary feature of Alzheimer's disease is a progressive decline in the ability to perform daily activities. This results from a gradually accumulating neuropathologic burden, which reduces the number of neurons and synapses. Impaired function of affected, but not yet dead, neurons may also contribute to diminished abilities in everyday life.

The neuropathology of AD is not randomly distributed in the brain. It primarily affects the hippocampus and related structures, as well as association areas of the cerebral cortex. Generally, the location of neuritic plaques correlates less well with cognition than do measures of neuronal loss and neurofibrillary tangle number.[1] Figure 1 depicts the accumulation of neurofibrillary tangles. This distribution leads to predictable areas of cognitive and behavioral disturbance that characterize the clinical syndrome of AD. Figure 2 illustrates typical behavioral functions associated with regions of the cerebral cortex. The pathologic distribution, therefore, predicts that AD will be associated with disturbances in memory, language, visual function, spatial processing, praxis, and behavioral control.

Although these functions will be individually addressed, clinicians must remember that intact cognition is seamless and that many overlaps exist between these aspects of human thought. An increasing sophistication and breadth of knowledge have emerged in the study of neuropsychologic deficits associated with AD. The primary literature on this topic is immense and complicated.

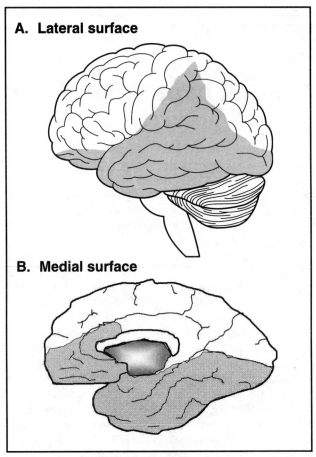

A. Lateral surface

B. Medial surface

Figure 1: Approximate distribution of highest neurofibrillary tangle counts from postmortem assessments.

This chapter reviews the typical phenomenology that is useful in clinical recognition and management of AD. More exhaustive reviews, which are precluded by space limitations here, may be found in Parks et al.[2]

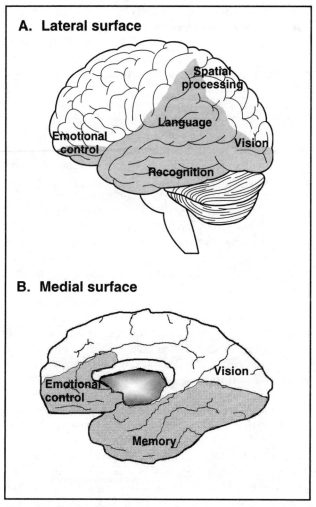

Figure 2: Cortical localization of cognitive and emotional ability (based on the effects of focal neurologic lesions) superimposed on neurofibrillary tangle distribution in the cortex of patients dying with AD.

Memory dysfunction is usually the first symptom recognized in AD. It is detectable by neuropsychologic tests even in preclinical phases of the disease.[3] The typical memory impairment in AD involves difficulties with learning new information but relative preservation of remote factual information.

Terms like *short-term memory loss* are often used to describe AD-related memory changes. Recent memories are impaired because new information cannot be adequately stored for later recall. Therefore, people affected by AD have difficulty remembering more recent events. It is important to recognize that there is not a fixed period of impaired recall. The span of the 'short term' is always increasing, because defective learning and storage of memories always progress once the problem begins. In most cases, learning is impaired well before overt memory symptoms, although old habits and preserved social skills may mask the problem. The type of information to be remembered also affects memory storage and recall. Declarative or factual memory systems allow us to store and recall specific information. These systems are responsible for humans' ability to remember that Abraham Lincoln was the 16th president of the United States. This is the memory type most impaired in AD. Procedural memory (ie, knowing how to perform some task) is often better preserved, which contributes to the superficial appearance of normality in mild AD. Emotional memories are often maintained as well, so that an AD patient may remember that a visit to a specific place, like the doctor's office or a day-care program, is unpleasant even if he or she cannot state why.

Because AD is a progressive illness, the character of memory loss and other cognitive impairments change over time. In the early (mild) and moderate stages of the illness, recall of remote material, learned before the onset of the mnemonic dysfunction, often appears to be preserved. However, detailed evaluations of patients indicate that deficits in recall of remote events are subtly present, particularly for specifics like dates and the timing of events.[4] In addition, generic knowledge, such as the number of days in a year, begins to be lost early in the disease course.[5] The breakdown in word-related memory and knowledge, also known as semantics, has a pervasive effect on cognition in AD, affecting broad areas of function, including language, motor skills (praxis), and visual processing. In the late stages of AD, memory dysfunction extends to complete failure of recall for previously well-remembered information, such as the names of the patient's own spouse or children.

Orientation

Closely associated with the breakdown of learning is progressive disorientation in time and place. Orientation requires a continuous process of updating memory systems with the passage of time and changes in location. Orientation to time is most vulnerable in early AD, and patients may dismiss deficiencies in this ability by stating that the day or date is not important to them, or that they have not looked at the news. For healthy older adults, such external sources of information are generally not required to maintain time and day orientation. More relative concepts of time can also be distorted, such that people with AD may be unable to recount the hour of the day, or the time passed since a recent holiday. As the illness progresses, orientation to place becomes more disrupted, and a person may become lost in familiar territory while driving or walking. Later, AD affects spatial orientation in the home, and individuals may not be able to navigate effectively indoors. This may be reported as confusion or difficulty in locating rooms. Spatial disorientation is often worse under conditions of low light, and can be particularly troublesome for families when the AD patient cannot find the bathroom. Loss of orientation to self is not typical, but severely affected patients can have language or response disturbances that prevent them from identifying themselves on questioning.

Language

Language impairments are a prominent part of the clinical picture of AD. They usually begin as word-finding difficulty in spontaneous speech and become evident as long pauses that interrupt the flow of speech. Patients will frequently describe a tip-of-the-tongue phenomenon when these gaps in their speech occur. Another manifestation of word-finding difficulty is circumlocution, in which the patient substitutes a series of descriptions or simpler words for the blocked one. For example, a person unable to find the word *lawnmower* might substitute the phrase, 'the red thing in the garage that's very loud and makes the grass shorter.' This phenomenon can be subtle and mistaken for verbal idiosyncrasies or mannerisms. It is sometimes necessary to confirm from family or other associates that the verbal pattern represents a change.

The language of the AD patient is usually vague. It frequently lacks specifics, substituting generic words or broad categories in place of more explicit nouns. Pronouns (eg, he, she, they) are often used in place of proper nouns. There is also an increased use of automatic phrases and clichés, particularly when the affected person is pressed for details. In addition, AD patients frequently have difficulty in naming actions.[6] Their descriptions of activities often substitute broader verbs, such as forms of 'be' or 'go,' in place of specific actions. On examination, impairment of object-naming ability often occurs, especially for parts of objects. This is referred to as anomia. The normal rhythm and melody of speech, known as prosody, may be lost and contributes to the bland nature of conversation in many AD patients. Prosody was affected in about one third of AD patients in one study.[7] Emotional intonations, known as affective prosody, were affected about twice as often. Unfortunately, as communication patterns become disrupted, problems in the care giving relationship arise.[8]

Impaired verbal comprehension becomes evident as AD progresses. Repetition is often preserved, even in more advanced cases. Longer phrases become more difficult for the AD patient to repeat, and the meaningfulness of the phrase has less impact on repetition ability than length.[9] This suggests that the problem is memory-span limitation, and not a breakdown in the language functions intrinsic to repeating phrases. Echolalia, or the tendency toward repeating all or part of another person's speech, occurs in some AD patients. It suggests a transcortical sensory aphasia, in which comprehension is disconnected from repetition. In late stages, progression to global aphasia or muteness (aphemia) is common.

Apraxia

Apraxia is a disorder of skilled movement despite intact strength and coordination. Nearly all AD patients will develop apraxia as the disease progresses, leading eventually to an inability to use eating utensils. The apraxia identified in most AD patients is an ideomotor disturbance, which means they have difficulty in translating an idea into the proper action. These problems reflect deficits in sensorimotor and spatiotemporal integration of motor plans.[10] A second form of apractic disturbance in AD represents a loss of the conceptual basis of tool use and mechanics, and is closely related to the loss of semantic knowledge underlying the language and memory problems in AD.[11] Another common manifestation of apraxia in AD is the inability to position parts of the body in space. This is a form of limb-kinetic apraxia, and can lead to problems in dressing. It also contributes to difficulties in positioning the body, eg, sitting in a chair.

Ideomotor apraxia in AD is similar to that observed after left parietal strokes, and often involves substituting a body part for the intended implement. On examination, the patient may demonstrate tooth-brushing by using his or her finger for the brush instead of grasping an imaginary handle. Difficulty integrating both hands into a bimanual task is a common early sign of apraxia in AD. For example, when affected persons are asked to

Table 1: Common Cognitive Findings in AD

Memory loss
- Deficit in learning
- Short-term memory loss
- Semantic knowledge failure

Disorientation
- Distorted time sense
- Spatial confusion

Aphasia
- Anomia
- Word-finding difficulty
- Vague, empty speech
- Poor comprehension

Apraxia
- Ideomotor apraxia
- Limb-kinetic apraxia

Complex visual dysfunction
- Agnosia
- Visuospatial impairment

Executive dysfunction
- Poor planning
- Poor judgment

Impaired abstract thought

Poor problem solving
- Disinhibition

Anosognosia
- Unawareness of impairment
- Denial of illness

demonstrate how they would slice a tomato, they often fail to hold the imagined vegetable. Another subtle sign of apraxia in AD is a compulsory verbalization, in which the patient can perform the task only by saying each step aloud. When asked to perform the task silently, these patients are often unable to do so. The reduced ability to think abstractly in AD may also be manifest during apraxia testing by the patient's need to act on an actual object, rather than an imagined one. When these people are asked to demonstrate how to strike a nail with a hammer, they will direct the action toward their leg or the examination table. When redirected to act in abstract space, apractic movements emerge.

Visual Abilities

Complex deficits in visual function are present in many AD patients, though only about half will complain of the problem or acknowledge it when questioned.[12] Visual function incorporates a broad spectrum of abilities. Depending on which tests are used to define visual performance, the frequency of deficits ranges from 0% to 100% of patients. Visual acuity is the most common screening test for vision, but it is normal in most AD patients. This contributes to underestimation of the importance of visual problems in AD patients. Furthermore, the visual difficulties evolve gradually and occur in individuals who may have problems verbally expressing subtle dysfunction. In addition, visual dysfunction is often misattributed to other, more overt cognitive problems. For instance, a patient with a disturbance in recognizing faces (prosopagnosia) is described as having 'forgotten' the faces of family members. In most circumstances, the degree of visual dysfunction is closely related to overall AD severity, but in some individuals, disturbances in complex visual function are the earliest signs of the disease.

Three broad categories of visual impairment have been observed in AD: impaired recognition (agnosia), impaired visuospatial processing, and impaired visual directed attention. Agnosia has many contributing factors in AD. At the most basic levels of visual processing, AD patients have impaired sensitivity to movement and visual contrast. Deficits in depth perception are also observed. Dysfunction in the visual association cortex may contribute to these problems, but it has a clearer role in other varieties of agnosia, such as prosopagnosia and visual object agnosia. In the latter, the ability to recognize an object visually is impaired. Interestingly, the individual may be able to describe its use, or even recognize it through other means, such as hearing or touching it.

Problems in spatial processing also occur, leading to spatial disorientation, such as becoming lost in an otherwise familiar environment. They may also manifest as difficulties with visual exploration, which has important implications for functional tasks, such as driving, that require active scanning of the environment. When severe, these deficits lead to a classically described visual disturbance known as Balint's syndrome. This is characterized by an inability to integrate bits of the spatial environment into a coherent, seamless whole. As a result, patients have difficulty using vision to guide hand and arm movements and to voluntarily direct their gaze toward items of interest.

Deficits in visual attention probably contribute to many of the visual and spatial disturbances in AD. Persons with AD are distractible. They are prone to involuntary redirections of visual attention when an event occurs away from where they are focusing. This contributes to impaired visuospatial problem solving, because the patient's attention is redirected to irrelevant information in the environment. This problem may contribute to AD patients' tendency to become lost because they are unable to maintain a consistent focus of attention. Also related to spatial processing disturbances, AD patients have problems in dividing their attention across multiple stimuli. This has relevance when persons affected by AD must sort through simultaneous, but spatially separated, information, such as directional signs in airports or on highways.

Executive or 'Frontal Lobe' Function

Problems with judgment, problem solving, planning, and abstract thought are common in AD. These behaviors require selecting tasks appropriately, sequencing their execution, and monitoring performance to ensure successful completion. Intact executive function also requires the suppression of inappropriate responses to the environment. Failures in this area of cognition are manifested as socially inappropriate behavior, disinhibition, and poor task persistence. Because of widely variable definitions of executive dysfunction and the absence of simple neuropsychologic tests for its diagnosis, the prevalence of these problems in AD is unclear. Detection of executive dysfunction is difficult in the presence of more severe focal cognitive deficits. Therefore, difficulties in regulating cognition and behavior tend to be most identifiable in the earlier stages of cognitive decline.

Self-Awareness

Many patients with AD do not recognize that they are impaired. This can range from mild denial to frank anosognosia (unawareness of illness). The problem has been linked to difficulty in implicit learning of intellectual limitations.[13] In effect, the patients forget that they forget things. They also forget *what* they forget, so when challenged by professionals or caregivers, persons affected by AD may seem surprised that others have recognized a problem. Similarly, AD patients underestimate their impairments across a broad spectrum of cognition and function. Some evidence supports a frontal-lobe basis for unawareness, and it is conceptually related to executive dysfunction.[14] The frequent concurrence of confabulation (ie, fabricating in place of remembering) with anosognosia supports this localization. Unawareness,

**Table 2: Common Noncognitive Findings
in Alzheimer's Disease**

Personality change
- Passive
- Self-centered
- Agitated/irritable

Apathy
- Hypoinitiation
- Poorly sustained effort

Depression

Anxiety
- Catastrophic reaction

Delusions
- Paranoia
- Misidentification

Hallucinations

Agitation
- Nonspecific motor behaviors
- Verbal aggression
- Physical aggression

Sleep disturbance
- Circadian shift
- Sleep inefficiency

when present, is an even greater source of distress to families than the overall disease severity.[15] As might be expected, depression occurs less often in AD patients with reduced self-awareness. Table 1 summarizes major cognitive features in AD.

Noncognitive Symptoms

Noncognitive or behavioral findings are common in AD and often account for a larger proportion of caregiver burden or stress than cognitive dysfunction. Typical noncognitive changes are listed in Table 2. Personality changes are common. Progressive passivity is the most frequent personality change early in the illness. Passive behavioral changes are seen in up to two thirds of patients with mild AD, along with increased self-centeredness. Agitation is seen in about one third of mildly affected patients.[16] Patients may also exhibit decreased emotional expression, diminished initiative, and decreased expressions of affection.[17] In many cases, passive personality change long predates cognitive abnormality, but this is only discerned retrospectively. One retrospective review suggested that social withdrawal, mood changes, or depression were present in more than 70% of cases, with a mean duration of more than 2 years before diagnosis of AD.[18]

Apathy

Apathy is a lack of motivation or behavioral initiation that is not attributable to disordered consciousness or emotional distress. Apathetic behaviors are often misattributed to a voluntary or willful refusal to cooperate. Caregivers may report experiences such as, 'I tell him to go do something, but he just sits there.' In such cases, it is important for the clinician to emphasize that the reduced initiative is usually not the result of volitional decision making, ie, it is not that the patient *won't* do as instructed, but rather that he or she *cannot* initiate the requested activity because of the disease. It can be difficult for clinicians and caregivers to distinguish the apathy of AD from depression, since both syndromes are associated with anhedonia and a reduction in self-initiated activities. Obtaining a sense of mood state from the patient can help with the distinction, because many patients can provide accurate self-assessment of mood well into the illness course.

Depression

Major or minor depression can be identified in up to half of AD patients.[19] Estimates of the frequency of major depression vary widely, ranging from about 5% to 25%. Much of the variability in reported prevalence represents methodologic differences and referral biases (eg, psychiatric vs neurologic clinic settings). Caregivers are about 3 times more likely to report depression than are the patients themselves. This may be due, in part, to the misattribution of withdrawal or apathy to the effects of depressed mood rather than dementia syndrome. Fortunately, AD patients are reliable reporters of their mood states on instruments like the Geriatric Depression Scale, even in moderate stages of dementia.[20] Unlike most symptoms associated with AD, depression does not increase with cognitive decline.[21]

The classic neurovegetative signs, such as weight loss, sleep disruption, and poor concentration, do not assist in the differentiation between apathy and depression because they are often present in dementia regardless of mood state. However, depression may magnify the cognitive deficits of AD through mechanisms such as reduced attention, poor concentration, and psychomotor slowing. Spells of mood-consistent tearfulness and verbalization of guilty feelings or fellings of worthlessness often help distinguish depression from apathy.

Anxiety is a common correlate of depression in AD patients. The anxiety tends to be more prominent in the earlier phases of the illness, and may be based on anticipation of potentially stressful circumstances or an adjustment reaction to the diagnosis of a dementing illness. A *catastrophic reaction* is an acute expression of overwhelming anxiety and fearfulness experienced by some AD patients, usually triggered by an adverse experience or in anticipation of one. These spells are typically brief, lasting less than 30 minutes, and self-limited.

Delusions

Delusions affect 30% to 50% of AD patients, according to most studies. The delusions are often paranoid in character and frequently include themes of theft, infidelity, and persecution. The prevalence of delusional thoughts increases with dementia severity, although they tend to persist if they occur earlier in the illness. Delusions are also closely associated with aggressive behavior.

Another common thought-content disorder in AD is delusional misidentification. Up to 30% of mild-to-moderate AD patients will misidentify important parts of their environment.[22] This may be evident as *Capgras' syndrome*, in which patients believe that caregivers or family members are impostors. Another common misidentification is when patients feel that their home is not their real home. Similarly, patients may be unable to identify themselves in mirrors. These kinds of misidentification are strongly associated with fearfulness and agitated behaviors. Patients with misidentification may also interpret television shows as being real or involving themselves or loved ones. Researchers have suggested that delusional misidentification results from the inability to continuously update memory with current information.[22]

Hallucinations

Hallucinations may occur in up to 25% of AD patients, but most studies suggest a frequency closer to 10% to 15%. They are typically visual but sometimes have auditory components. Frequent themes include seeing deceased parents or siblings, unknown intruders (especially children or 'little people'), and animals.[12] Typically, the hallucinations are not threatening. Misperceptions also occur, and may represent the combined effect of disordered visual function and thought content (eg, a shrub in the dimly lit yard is perceived as a potential intruder). Generally, hallucinations are less predictive of agitation and aggression than are delusions.

Agitation and Sundowning

Agitation is an exceptionally common complaint of caregivers in AD, with reported frequencies of 50% to 60%. Unfortunately, the term *agitation* does not represent a specific symptom. Therefore, it requires careful description to identify the specific behavioral patterns and to plan a therapeutic approach. Agitation can be divided into several behaviors:

(1) physical aggression/assaultiveness
(2) verbal aggression/outbursts
(3) physical nonaggressive behaviors[23]

Sundowning is a colloquial term for predictable increases in confusion and behavioral symptoms in the afternoon and evening hours. Although this behavior pattern occurs in up to 25% of AD patients, it also is not a discrete symptom and represents diurnal variation rather than a specific pathophysiology.

Aggressive behaviors are most clearly linked to delusions and delusional misidentification. In one series, more than 80% of patients with frequent aggression (>1 episode per month) had delusions.[24] Verbal aggression is more common than physical assault. Men and patients with more advanced functional decline are more prone to physical or verbal aggression. Aggressive behaviors usually follow an escalating pattern, with verbal outbursts preceding the physical acts. Caregiver assistance with personal care, especially bathing, is a typical provocation for aggression.

Wandering, pacing, and recurrent purposeless activities are typical nonaggressive motor behaviors. Wandering is often triggered by delusional misidentification, in that the affected person may be trying to locate his or her 'real' home or locate a 'missing' loved one. Wandering has also been associated with poor visuospatial abilities, perhaps reflecting difficulty with incorporating visual information into a coherent spatial map. As such, dim light or nighttime can be exacerbating factors for wanderers. Risks resulting from wandering include getting lost outdoors, with its consequent hazard of exposure-related morbidity, as well as an increased likelihood of fractures. Pacing is somewhat more idiosyncratic, with fewer clearly associated neuropsychologic features. The near-ceaseless pacing of some AD patients contributes to accelerated weight loss, which can be refractory to dietary interventions unless the locomotor activity is reduced. A more benign form of physical nonaggressive behavior is rummaging in drawers or closets. Patients who do this appear to be searching for some item, but are often unable to describe what it is. This frequent sorting of personal effects is also associated with delusions of theft.

Sleep Disturbance

Subtle changes in sleep patterns are detectable early in the course of AD. These include increased time awake and increased nocturnal awakenings.[25] Progressive breakdown of circadian rhythms can be identified as the disease progresses. As a result, many patients will exhibit increased daytime napping. This sleep is often of poor quality, not reaching stage 3 or 4 (slow wave) sleep. Patients may spend more time in bed, but sleep efficiency is poor. Fatigue associated with functional sleep deprivation can also increase irritability and confusion. The degree of sleep disturbance is associated with both the amount of daytime behavioral problems and overall disease severity. Behavioral disturbances associated with disturbed sleep can be further exacerbated by irritability in caregivers, which increases with interruption of their sleep to provide care or comfort to the patient.

Changes in the Neurologic Examination

Throughout most of its course, AD spares the elemental neurologic examination. In later stages, gait disturbances and extrapyramidal signs, such as rigidity, become prominent. Gait disorders typically begin as hesitancy and fearfulness, and progress to a need for a widened base of support, decreased stride length, and increased lateral sway. The latter has both apractic and ataxic components and has been called a *frontal gait disturbance*. Not surprisingly, the prevalence of gait disorder is increased in patients showing other frontal lobe signs, such as pathologic snout and grasp reflexes. Rigidity and stooped posture have been identified in more than 40% of patients in some AD series, but in many, this represents the effects of antipsychotic drug treatment. Perhaps as a consequence of gait disturbances, falls are 3 times more common among severely impaired AD patients than in the general population.[26] Seizures have been reported in 10% to 20% of AD patients, again often late in the disease. They are frequently associated with a period of more rapid worsening of symptoms. Myoclonus, consisting of brisk, irregular muscle contractions, occurs in 5% to 10% of AD patients. Multifocal myoclonus can be difficult to distinguish from seizures in later-stage patients, and may account for the apparent frequency of seizures.

The primary sensory examination is usually unremarkable, but subtle deficits may be present. Attention difficulties complicate sensory system examination in many AD patients. As a result, attention-dependent testing, such as for visual fields and auditory discrimination, is frequently abnormal. These abnormalities are more often a reflection of cognitive impairment rather than true deficits in primary sensory abilities. One possible exception is olfactory function. Several studies suggest that AD patients are impaired in odor detection, but the ability of olfactory testing to discriminate AD from other age-related illnesses is controversial.

Course and Staging

AD is defined by its progressive nature. The average duration of illness is about 8 years,[27] though the range is wide and depends on many factors, including age at onset and general health. For patients with younger onset and good general health, 8 years is often an underestimate. A better prediction is that life expectancy will be halved. Nearly all aspects of cognition, behavior, and function become progressively more impaired over the years of

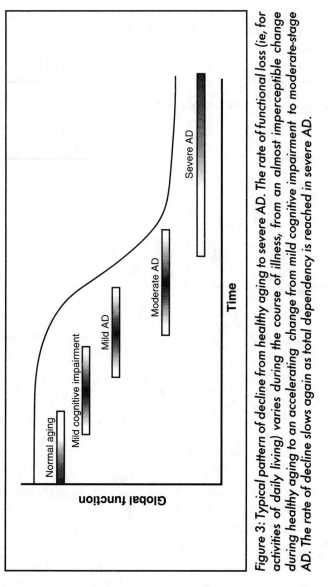

Figure 3: Typical pattern of decline from healthy aging to severe AD. The rate of functional loss (ie, for activities of daily living) varies during the course of illness, from an almost imperceptible change during healthy aging to an accelerating change from mild cognitive impairment to moderate-stage AD. The rate of decline slows again as total dependency is reached in severe AD.

Table 3: Clinical Dementia Rating*

	Memory	Orientation	Judgment and Problem Solving
None (0)	No memory loss or slight, inconsistent forgetfulness	Fully oriented	Solves everyday problems well; judgment good in relation to past performance
Questionable (0.5)	Consistent slight forgetfulness; partial recollection of events; 'benign' forgetfulness	Fully oriented except for slight difficulty with time relationships	Slight impairment in solving problems, similarities, differences
Mild (1)	Moderate memory loss; more marked for recent events; defect interferes with everyday activities	Moderate difficulty with time relationships; oriented for place at examination; may have geographic disorientation elsewhere	Moderate difficulty in handling problems, similarities, differences; social judgment usually maintained

*Adapted from Hughes, et al[30]

Community Affairs	Home and Hobbies	Personal Care
Independent function at usual level in job, shopping, business, and financial affairs, volunteer and social groups	Life at home, hobbies, intellectual interests well maintained	Fully capable of self-care
Slight impairment in these activities	Life at home, hobbies, intellectual interests slightly impaired	Fully capable of self-care
Unable to function independently at these activities, though may still be engaged in some; appears normal to casual inspection	Mild but definite impairment of function at home; more difficult chores abandoned; more complicated hobbies and interests abandoned	Needs prompting

(continued on next page)

Table 3: Clinical Dementia Rating (continued)

	Memory	Orientation	Judgment and Problem Solving
Moderate (2)	Severe memory loss; only highly learned material retained; new material rapidly lost	Severe difficulty with time relationships; usually disoriented in time, often to place	Severely impaired in handling problems, similarities, differences; social judgment usually impaired
Severe (3)	Severe memory loss; only fragments remain	Oriented to person only	Unable to make judgments or solve problems

the illness. There is, however, much interindividual variability in expression, such that no 2 patients will share exactly the same clinical course. Age, gender, general health, genetics, culture, and social situation also have major impacts on the way that AD is expressed. A general rule is that whatever cognitive symptoms occur first will continue to be the worst (ie, relatively most severe) throughout the illness course. With the exception of depressive symptoms, noncognitive aspects of the illness also inevitably worsen, at least until the patient lacks the physi-

Community Affairs	Home and Hobbies	Personal Care
No pretense of independent function outside home; appears well enough to be taken to functions outside family home	Only simple chores preserved; very restricted interests, poorly sustained	Requires assistance in dressing, hygiene, keeping of personal effects
No pretense of independent function outside home; appears too ill to be taken to functions outside family home	No significant function in home	Requires much help with personal care; frequent incontinence

cal ability to express the disturbed behavior. Functional decline is nonlinear, with the greatest rate of decline in moderately affected individuals. The typical course follows an inverted S-curve (Figure 3).[28] Plateaux (periods of stability in cognitive symptoms) may indicate a more benign overall course of the illness.[29] Patients will lose complex instrumental activities of daily living (IADL), such as financial management, home maintenance, or meal preparation, earlier than basic activities of daily living (ADL), like bathing, toileting, or feeding.

Table 4: Global Deterioration Scale[35]

Stage 1: No Cognitive Decline
Clinical phase: Normal

Characteristics:
- No subjective complaints of memory deficit. No memory deficit on clinical interview

Stage 2: Very Mild Cognitive Decline
Clinical phase: Forgetfulness

Characteristics:
- Subjective complaints of memory deficit, most frequently forgetting where one has placed familiar objects and names one formerly knew well
- No objective evidence of memory deficit on clinical interview
- No objective deficits in employment or social situations
- Appropriate concern with respect to symptomology

Stage 3: Mild Cognitive Decline
Clinical phase: Early confusion

Characteristics:
- Earliest clear-cut deficits. Manifestations in more than 1 of the following areas:
  - Patient may have gotten lost when traveling to an unfamiliar location
  - Coworkers become aware of patient's relatively poor performance
  - Work and name-finding deficits become evident to intimates

- Patient may read a passage or a book and retain relatively little material
- Patient may demonstrate decreased faculty in remembering names when introduced to new people
- Patient may have lost or misplaced an object of value
- Concentration deficit may be evident on clinical testing

Stage 4: Moderate Cognitive Decline
Clinical phase: Late confusion

Characteristics: Clear-cut deficit on careful clinical interview

- Deficits manifest in following areas:
  - Decreased knowledge of current and recent events
  - May exhibit some deficit in memory of personal history
  - Concentration deficit elicited on serial subtractions
  - Decreased ability to travel, handle finances, etc

- Frequently, no deficit in following areas:
  - Orientation to time and person
  - Recognition of familiar persons and faces
  - Ability to travel to familiar areas

- Inability to perform complex tasks

- Denial is the dominant defense mechanism

- Flattening of affect and withdrawal from challenging situations occur

(continued on next page)

Table 4: Global Deterioration Scale[35] (continued)

Stage 5: Moderately Severe Cognitive Decline
Clinical phase: Early dementia

Characteristics:

- Patients can no longer survive without some assistance

- Patients are unable during interview to recall a major relevant aspect of their current lives (eg, the names of close members of their family, such as grandchildren; the name of the high school or college from which they graduated; etc)

- Frequently, some disorientation to time (date, day of week, season, etc) or to place

- An educated person may have difficulty counting back from 40 by 4's or 20 by 2's

- Persons at this stage retain knowledge of many major facts about themselves and others. They invariably know their own names and generally know their spouse's and children's names. They require no assistance in toileting and eating, but may have some difficulty choosing the proper clothes to wear

Stage 6: Severe Cognitive Decline
Clinical phase: Middle dementia

Characteristics:

- May occasionally forget the name of the spouse upon whom they are entirely dependent for survival

- Will be largely unaware of all recent events and experiences in their lives

- Retain some knowledge of their past lives, but very sketchy
- Generally unaware of their surroundings, the year, the season, etc
- May have difficulty counting from 10, both backward and sometimes forward
- Will require assistance with the activities of daily living (eg, may become incontinent, will require travel assistance, but occasionally, will display ability to travel to familiar locations)
- Diurnal rhythm frequently disturbed
- Almost always recall their own name
- Frequently continue to be able to distinguish familiar from unfamiliar persons in their environment
- Personality and emotional changes occur. These are quite variable and include:
  - Delusional behavior (eg, patients may accuse their spouse of being an impostor, may talk to imaginary figures in the environment, or to their own reflection in the mirror)
  - Obsessive symptoms (eg, person may continually repeat simple cleaning activities)
  - Anxiety symptoms, agitation, and even previously nonexistent violent behavior may occur
  - Cognitive abulia (ie, loss of willpower, because an individual cannot carry a thought long enough to determine a purposeful course of action)

(continued on next page)

Table 4: Global Deterioration Scale[35] (continued)

Stage 7: Very Severe Cognitive Decline
Clinical phase: Late dementia

Characteristics:

- All verbal abilities are lost. Frequently, there is no speech at all—only grunting

- Incontinent of urine; requires assistance toileting and feeding

- Loss of basic psychomotor skills (eg, ability to walk). The brain appears to no longer be able to tell the body what to do

- Generalized and cortical neurologic signs and symptoms are frequently present

Pfeffer RI, et al: *J Gerontol* 1982;37:323-329 Copyright© The Gerontological Society of America. Reproduced by permission of the publisher.

Staging

Families often express interest in knowing the *stage* of the illness. While the wide variability in clinical expression makes staging difficult, several staging schemes have evolved and offer some clinical utility. The greatest value of these systems is in quantitative ranking of illness severity for research functions. The Clinical Dementia Rating (CDR) (Table 3) is a scale that uses a structured interview format to assess 6 domains of cognition and function.[30] Ratings in the 6 domains are then used to assign categories of mild, moderate, and severe decline. The scale was subsequently expanded to include more globally defined categories of *profound* and *terminal* dementia. Several scoring algorithms have been

Table 5: Clinical Staging of AD

Mild
- Impaired memory, excused or covered
- Insidious losses in instrumental ADL
- Preserved basic ADL
- Subtle personality change
- Socially normal

Moderate
- Obvious memory impairment
- Overt instrumental ADL impairment
- Basic ADL failing
- Prominent behavioral difficulties
- Social skills variable
- Needs supervision

Severe
- Memory fragments only
- Does not recognize familiar people
- Needs assistance with basic ADL
- Fewer troublesome behaviors (usually)
- Reduced mobility

implemented and allow flexibility in applying the scale.[31] While generally useful, the scale lacks explicit means of weighing nonmemory cognitive symptoms, such as aphasia, apraxia, or visuospatial dysfunction. Similarly, the role of mood and behavioral changes must be incorporated in the ratings of several domains. Nonetheless, the CDR is a standard for reporting global severity in clinical trials and other research reports.

The Global Deterioration Scale (GDS) (Table 4) is a 7-level scale, ranging from a score of 1, which represents no cognitive decline, to 7, indicating very severe impairment.[32] The GDS is based on empiric observations of typical symptom and behavior clusters. The validity of the individual clusters has been questioned because many patients have symptoms that span 2 or 3 of the stages. This makes the clinician's assignment of the stage dependent on a global sense, even if there are examples of behavior that fall outside the assigned stage. In addition, the implication that dementia is not present until stage 3 is problematic if the individual otherwise meets criteria for dementia (see Chapter 4). Nonetheless, the scale provides reliable and valid global information. It can be used in conjunction with the Functional Assessment Staging (FAST)[33] instrument to provide more explicit measures of function. The 7 levels of the GDS can be cumbersome and difficult for families to interpret. Broad categories like mild (GDS = 2 to 3), moderate (GDS = 4 to 5), and severe (GDS = 6 to 7) are sufficiently informative for most routine staging.

In clinical use, mild dementia might be thought of as mildly limiting independence for complex parts of daily function. Though memory and orientation difficulties exist, they may be subtle and go unnoticed except by those closest to the affected person. By the moderate stage, overt confusion and other cognitive and behavioral signs are present and the person typically requires significant assistance with IADLs. In the severe stage, dementia is evident to casual observers and support is needed for ADLs as well. Only fragments of memory are retained. Many individuals with AD are institutionalized as they move through the later years of the illness. The severe phase of the illness often lasts for several years. Typical considerations for staging are shown in Table 5. Mortality is increased significantly for persons with AD. Immobility and cachexia are common in later phases of the illness. More than 75% of Alzheimer's patients who become nonambulatory also develop significant, often multiple, painful joint contractures.[34] The most common causes of death attributable to end-stage AD are pneumonia, urinary infections, decubitus ulcers, malnutrition, and dehydration.

References

1. Bierer LM, Hof PR, Purohit DP, et al: Neocortical neurofibrillary tangles correlate with dementia severity in Alzheimer's disease. *Arch Neurol* 1995;52:81-88.

2. Parks RW, Zec RF, Wilson RS, eds: *Neuropsychology of Alzheimer's Disease and Other Dementias.* New York, Oxford University Press, 1993.

3. Jacobs DM, Sano M, Dooneief G, et al: Neuropsychological detection and characterization of preclinical Alzheimer's disease. *Neurology* 1995;45:957-962.

4. Storandt M, Kaskie B, Von Dras DD, et al: Temporal memory for remote events in healthy aging and dementia. *Psychol Aging* 1998;13:4-7.

5. Norton LE, Bondi MW, Salmon DP, et al: Deterioration of generic knowledge in patients with Alzheimer's disease: evidence from the Number Information Test. *J Clin Exp Neuropsychol* 1997;19:857-866.

6. Cappa SF, Binetti G, et al: Object and action naming in Alzheimer's disease and frontotemporal dementia. *Neurology* 1998;50:351-355.

7. Perez Trullen JM, Modrego Pardo PJ: Comparative study of aprosody in Alzheimer's disease and in multi-infarct dementia. *Dementia* 1996;7:59-62.

8. Ripich D, Vertes D, Whitehouse P, et al: Turn-taking and speech act patterns in the discourse of senile dementia of the Alzheimer's type patient. *Brain Lang* 1991;40:330-343.

9. Bayles KA, Tomoeda CK, et al: Phrase repetition in Alzheimer's disease. *Brain Lang* 1996;54:246-261.

10. Benke T: Two forms of apraxia in Alzheimer's disease. *Cortex* 1993;29:715-725.

11. Ochipa C, Rothi LJ, Heilman KM: Conceptual apraxia in Alzheimer's disease. *Brain* 1992;115:1061-1071.

12. Mendez MF, Mendez MA, Martin R, et al: Complex visual disturbances in Alzheimer's disease. *Neurology* 1990;40:439-443.

13. Starkstein SE, Sabe L, Cuerva AG, et al: Anosognosia and procedural learning in Alzheimer's disease. *Neuropsychiatry Neuropsychol Behav Neurol* 1997;10:96-101.

14. Patterson MB, Mack JL, et al: Executive functions and Alzheimer's disease: problems and prospects. *Eur J Neurol* 1996;3:15.

15. Seltzer B, Vasterling JJ, Yoder JA, et al: Awareness of deficit in Alzheimer's disease: relation to caregiver burden. *Gerontologist* 1997;37:20-24.

16. Rubin EH, Morris JC, Berg L: The progression of personality changes in senile dementia of the Alzheimer's type. *J Am Geriatr Soc* 1987;35:721-725.

17. Mendez MF, Martin RJ, Smyth KA, et al: Psychiatric symptoms associated with Alzheimer's disease. *J Neuropsychiatry Clin Neurosci* 1990;2:28-33.

18. Jost BC, Grossberg GT: The evolution of psychiatric symptoms in Alzheimer's disease: a natural history study. *J Am Geriatr Soc* 1996;44:1078-1081.

19. Lyketsos CG, Steele C, Baker L, et al: Major and minor depression in Alzheimer's disease: prevalence and impact. *J Neuropsychiatry Clinic Neurosci* 1997;9:556-561.

20. Katz IR: Diagnosis and treatment of depression in patients with Alzheimer's disease and other dementias. *J Clin Psychiatry* 1998;59:38-44.

21. Cooper JK, Mungas D, Weiler PG, et al: Relation of cognitive status and abnormal behaviors in Alzheimer's disease. *J Am Geriatr Soc* 1990;38:867-870.

22. Forstl H, Besthorn C, Burns A, et al: Delusional misidentification in Alzheimer's disease: a summary of clinical and biological aspects. *Psychopathology* 1994;27:194-199.

23. Deutsch LH, Rovner BW: Agitation and other noncognitive abnormalities in Alzheimer's disease. *Psychiatr Clin North Am* 1991;14:341-351.

24. Gilley DW, Wilson RS, Beckett LA, et al: Psychotic symptoms and physically aggressive behavior in Alzheimer's disease. *J Am Geriatr Soc* 1997;45:1074-1079.

25. Vitiello MV, Prinz PN, Williams DE, et al: Sleep disturbances in patients with mild-stage Alzheimer's disease. *J Gerontol* 1990; 45:M131-M138.

26. Buchner DM, Larson EB: Falls and fractures in patients with Alzheimer-type dementia. *JAMA* 1987;257:1492-1495.

27. Jost BC, Grossberg GT: The natural history of Alzheimer's disease: a brain bank study. *J Am Geriatr Soc* 1995;43:1248-1255.

28. Stern Y, Liu X, Albert M, et al: Application of a growth curve approach to modeling the progression of Alzheimer's disease. *J Gerontol A Biol Sci Med Sci* 1996;51:M179-M184.

29. Piccini C, Bracco L, Falcini M, et al: Natural history of Alzheimer's disease: prognostic value of plateaux. *J Neurol Sci* 1995;131:177-182.

30. Hughes CP, Berg L, Danzinger WL, et al: A new clinical scale for the staging of dementia. *Br J Psychiatry* 1982;140:566-572.

31. Fillenbaum GG, Peterson B, Morris JC: Estimating the validity of the Clinical Dementia Rating Scale: the CERAD experience. Consortium to Establish a Registry for Alzheimer's Disease. *Aging* 1996;8:379-385.

32. Reisberg B, Ferris SH, de Leon MJ, et al: The Global Deterioration Scale for assessment of primary degenerative dementia. *Am J Psychiatry* 1982;139:1136-1139.

33. Sclan SG, Reisberg B: Functional Assessment Staging (FAST) in Alzheimer's disease: reliability, validity, and ordinality. *Int Psychogeriatr* 1992;4:55-69.

34. Souren LE, Franssen EH, Reisberg B: Contractures and loss of function in patients with Alzheimer's disease. *J Am Geriatr Soc* 1995;43:650-655.

35. Reisberg B: Clinical presentation, diagnosis, and symptomatology of age-associated cognitive decline and Alzheimer's disease. In: *Alzheimer's Disease: The Standard Reference*. New York, Free Press, 1983, pp 173-187.

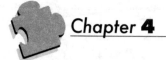

Chapter **4**

Clinical Expression of Other Progressive Dementing Illnesses

U ntil recently, investigators placed little emphasis on the differences in clinical expressions of the many causes of dementia. Consequently, few clinicians expressed much interest in extensive differential diagnosis beyond the exclusion of the traditional, but rare, reversible dementias such as neurosyphilis or vitamin B_{12} deficiency. However, even among the irreversible dementing illnesses, accurate diagnosis is essential to initiate appropriate treatments, to provide information about prognosis, and to discuss factors that may affect the illness's course. Accurate diagnosis is also needed to adequately counsel families about heritable risks and to determine the utility of genetic testing. As more effective treatments and interventions become available through the intense research efforts now underway, clinical differential diagnosis in dementia will become even more important.

Cognitive Changes With Aging

There is universal agreement that losses in thinking and memory occur with the healthy aging process, but the description and clinical implications of those losses are controversial. Age-Associated Memory Impairment (AAMI) and Aging-Associated Cognitive Decline (AACD) are classifications of age-related cognitive change that typically involve reports of memory impairment accompanied by mild changes on objective memory testing and slowed information processing. These categories are principally useful for research classification and their clinical utility is undemonstrated.

AAMI and AACD have been considered to carry a benign prognosis, but more recent evidence suggests that this may not be case.[1]

AAMI is characterized by subjective memory complaints arising in patients after 50 years of age with neuropsychologic scores more than one standard deviation below the norm for young adults on memory tests.[2]

AACD includes insidious onset of cognitive decline at least 6 months in duration, and impairment in memory, language, attention, concentration, thinking, or visual functioning. Scores on standardized neuropsychologic testing should be at least one standard deviation below age-corrected norms in at least one of these realms. The impairment does not significantly reduce daily function, and is generally not progressive.[3] Prevalence rates vary widely with the methods and criteria used to study the problem. About 25% of the older adult population has findings consistent with AAMI.[4]

Mild Cognitive Impairment

Another way of categorizing late-life cognitive decline is known as mild cognitive impairment (MCI). Although several subtypes of MCI have been described,[5] the term is usually used in reference to the *amnestic form* of MCI. In this variant, the bedside findings are typically restricted to memory, but unlike AACD, the deficits are clearly evident on bedside testing. Amnestic MCI may represent an incipient stage of dementia, since about 50% of individuals affected with a pure amnestic form of MCI will progress into dementia, usually Alzheimer's disease, over a 3- to 5-year period. Current practice guidelines suggest serial and systematic follow-up of these patients to determine whether the condition is progressing toward Alzheimer's disease.[6] Recommended sources of information in the systematic follow-up include family reports, bedside instruments such as the MMSE, or neuropsychologic testing. Simple reassurance without evaluation (eg, "Don't worry about it. You're just getting old like the rest of us.") is inappropriate.

The MCI category has been criticized for a lack of validity, consistency, and predictive value.[7] While it is clear that all progressive dementia must pass through an incipient phase, the alternative argument that all mild cognitive impairments will progress to dementia very much depends on the definitions used. This is perhaps most clear for cognitive impairments associated with cerebrovascular disease. A clinical state known as vascular cognitive impairment with no dementia (VCIND) has been described in these patients. VCIND is associated with a high risk for mortality (>50%), but in one study, less than half of the patients followed developed dementia over a 5-year follow-up period.[8]

Dementia vs Depression

The differential diagnosis of degenerative dementia vs cognitive impairment resulting from depression can be difficult. In depression, the patient often complains of cognitive difficulties. In dementia, it is usually a relative who brings the patient to the physician. The duration of depression is often shorter, measured in weeks or a few months, and it typically has a more discrete onset than most causes of dementia. A personal or family history of depression also increases the likelihood of depression as a cause of cognitive difficulty. It is unusual for first-ever depression to present after the age of 60 in the absence of a clear precipitant such as grieving. Confirming mood changes with the patient is important, because families will often report depression based on observations of dementia-induced apathy. In addition to, or instead of, reporting low mood, depressed patients will be more likely to express feelings of diminished self-worth. Patients with

Table 1: Features Useful in Differentiating Delirium, Depression, and Dementia

	Delirium	Depression	Dementia
Onset	acute	recognized	insidious
Duration	hours-days	weeks-months	months-years
Complainant	varies	patient	family
Consciousness	clouded*	clear, but slow	clear*

* Mandatory for diagnosis

depression also typically demonstrate psychomotor slowing, and they produce incomplete answers with poor effort on testing (eg, "I don't know"). Even when a patient's cognitive function improves with treatment of depression, there is nearly a 50% risk for developing irreversible dementia over the next several years.[9]

Dementia vs Delirium

Dementia must be differentiated from delirium in the older adult. Delirium is almost always an acute, reversible, and metabolically induced state of fluctuating consciousness. Focal neurologic causes are identified in less than 10% of delirium in older patients, leading many neurologists to use the term *metabolic encephalopathy* synonymously with delirium. The distinction between delirium and dementia may be hindered by the fact that delirium is a common complication of chronic dementia.

Medications are the most common cause of reversible cognitive impairment. Any drug (including alcohol) that affects systemic homeostasis or neuronal function must be considered a possible contributing factor to abnormal behavior or cognitive impairment. If drugs are suspected, they then should be eliminated or substituted to assess for cognitive side effects. Other common causes of delirium in the elderly are fluid and electrolyte derangement, cerebral hypoperfusion, pain, and infections. Features useful for differentiating delirium, dementia, and depression are listed in Table 1.

Non-Alzheimer Dementias

Diagnostic and Statistical Manual of Mental Disorders, 4th edition (DSM-IV) criteria for dementia require the presence of memory deficits, but many non-Alzheimer dementias can have subtle or no memory deficits. Cummings and Benson[10] suggested an alternative diagnostic scheme to accommodate the variable expression of memory deficits in these less common dementia syndromes. Their approach does not require memory impairment to define dementia, but rather depends on identifying impairment in at least 3 of the following functions: language, memory, visuospatial skills, emotion/personality, or higher-level cognitive functions (abstraction, calculation, judgment, executive function). In further contrast to DSM-IV, these guidelines do not require cognitive impairment to be severe enough to interfere with social or occupational function. This is especially pertinent among the illnesses discussed later in this chapter because many include motor dysfunction. Differentiating motor from cognitive sources of functional disability in these illnesses can be challenging. Despite the clinical utility of the Cummings and Benson approach for non-Alzheimer causes of dementia, clinicians must recognize that no large-scale validation exists of their guidelines. This chapter will discuss illnesses that, like AD, include dementia as part of the presenting complaint and therefore may need to be considered in the differential diagnosis of the person with cognitive decline or behavioral change.

Dementia with Lewy Bodies

Dementia associated with atypical clinical or neuropathologic manifestations of Parkinson's disease (PD) is increasingly recognized. The nomenclature on this topic has been very confused, but a consensus conference in 1995 recommended use of the term dementia with Lewy bodies (DLB) to supersede a myriad of other descriptors, including Diffuse Lewy Body Disease, Lewy Body Variant of Alzheimer's disease, Alzheimer's/Parkinson's complex, and parkinsonian dementia.

Lewy bodies are spherical intracytoplasmic neuronal inclusion bodies composed primarily of neurofilament material. F.H. Lewy first recognized them as markers for PD in 1912. In both PD and DLB, Lewy bodies are found in the brain stem, thalamus, and basal ganglia. But in DLB, Lewy bodies are also extensively found in the cerebral cortex. Concomitant expression of the pathologic markers of AD, particularly neuritic plaques, is observed in 50% to 75% of cases. There is a historical justice in the use of Lewy's name to label this spectrum of illness. By 1923, Lewy recognized that most patients with Parkinson's type motor dysfunction had significant cognitive deficits. Parkinson had overlooked this feature in his original description of the *shaking palsy* in 1817.

Clinical Expression

DLB can be considered dementia with signs of cortical dysfunction accompanied by findings suggesting parkinsonism on history or examination. It typically follows a progressive course similar to AD, but some cases evolve rapidly and can be confused with Creutzfeldt-Jakob disease (CJD).

Key elements of the criteria[11] are shown in Table 2. These criteria offer high specificity (90% to 100%) but relatively poor sensitivity (50% to 60%).[12]

Cognitive and Behavioral Findings

The cognitive/behavioral and parkinsonian signs typically evolve within 1 year of each other. Visual hallucinations and mild delusions are frequently evident early in the course and may be provoked or exacerbated by treatment

Table 2: Key Elements of the Criteria for Diagnosing Senile Dementia of Lewy Body Type

I.   Fluctuating cognitive impairment affecting both memory and higher cortical functions characterized by:

- Declines in language, visuospatial ability, praxis, or reasoning skills are common

- Fluctuation (including both episodic confusion and lucid intervals) may be evident:

    1. On cognitive testing, and/or
    2. By variable performance in daily living skills

II. At least one of the following should be present:

- Visual and/or auditory hallucinations (usually accompanied by secondary paranoid delusions)

- Mild extrapyramidal features, occurring:

    1. Spontaneously, or
    2. With neuroleptic medication

- Repeated episodes of:

    1. Unexplained falls, and/or
    2. Transient clouding or loss of consciousness

III. Clinical features persist over weeks, months, or longer

IV. Progressive illness, leading to severe dementia

V.   No underlying illness accounts for the fluctuation

VI. No cerebral vascular disease, ie,

- No history of confirmed stroke, and

- No evidence of significant cerebral ischemic damage on examination or imaging

Abstracted from McKeith et al[11]

Table 3: Typical Elements of Executive Function Impairment

These fall into broad categories that can be thought of as resulting in (1) losses of normal function, or (2) pathologic behaviors superimposed on the normal behaviors. Patients may simultaneously or alternately express behaviors from both categories.

Functional loss

- Impersistence
- Impaired problem solving
- Loss of initiative and self-direction
- Loss of motivation
- Poor planning
- Social withdrawal

Added behavior

- Disinhibition
- Distractibility
- Impulsivity
- Perseveration
- Social impropriety
- Tangentiality

of the parkinsonism. Disorders of executive function, which is the ability to plan and initiate appropriate behaviors, are among the earliest cognitive problems. Executive function impairments are fundamentally important in many of the non-Alzheimer dementias. Key components of executive function are listed in Table 3. Cortical findings, especially apraxia and visuospatial disturbances, are often prominent. Other changes include general slowness of thought and

Table 4: Vascular Disorders Leading to Dementia

Hemorrhage

- Intracerebral
  - hypertension
  - amyloid angiopathy
- Extracerebral
  - aneurysmal (or other subarachnoid) bleeding
  - subdural hematoma
- Posthemorrhagic hydrocephalus

Hypoperfusion

- Cardiac arrest
- Sustained hypotension

Ischemic stroke

- Large emboli—cortical predominance
  - artery-to-artery
  - cardiogenic

    ‡ acute MI

    ‡ atrial fibrillation
- Recurrent small emboli—subcortical predominance
  - endocarditis
  - atrial myxoma

---

action (bradyphrenia or psychomotor slowing). Apathy and depression are also frequent.

Physical Findings

Tremor is not a major feature of the parkinsonism in most cases of DLB. Rigidity is far more typical, affecting about 75% of cases. Bradykinesia also appears in most cases. Transient and otherwise unexplained lapses of conscious-

- In situ thrombosis—subcortical predominance
  - lacunar infarction
- Nonspecific vasculopathy—subcortical predominance
  - subacute arteriosclerotic encephalopathy (Binswanger's disease)

Postsurgical

- Post-CABG syndrome
- Fat emboli
- Air emboli

Vasculitis

- Autoimmune vasculitides
  - systemic (eg, lupus)
  - CNS (eg, granulomatous angiitis)
- Infectious vasculitides
  - neurosyphilis
  - Lyme disease

ness can be easily mistaken for seizures or orthostatic syncope. Unsteady gait and postural instability are typical.

Epidemiology

DLB probably represents the second most common form of degenerative dementia, accounting for 15% to 25% of cases.[13] Men are affected about twice as often as women. Onset of DLB is rare before age 55 to 60.

Table 5: Key Elements for Diagnosing Vascular Dementia

Clinical diagnosis of vascular dementia ideally includes:

I. Evidence for a dementia syndrome including:

- Memory dysfunction
- Evidence for other cognitive or behavioral deficits, which may include:
    - executive dysfunction
    - focal cortical signs (eg, aphasia, apraxia, or agnosia)
    - personality changes (eg, apathy or irritability)
    - affective changes (eg, depression or anxiety)

II. Evidence for cerebrovascular disease, supported by at least one of the following:

- History of clear-cut cerebrovascular events (eg, acute hemiparesis, sudden diplopia)
- Physical findings consistent with cerebrovascular events (eg, Babinski's sign, asymmetric hyperreflexia)
- Imaging findings consistent with clinically relevant cerebrovascular events, eg:
    - two or more discrete infarcts outside the cerebellum
    - white matter disease exceeding 25% of white matter volume

Vascular Dementia

Cerebral ischemia has long been considered a primary cause of dementia. However, experimental evidence does not support theories that chronic cerebral oxygen depri-

III. Evidence that I and II are temporally linked (eg, one of the following):

- No evidence for cognitive decline prior to stroke episode
- Abrupt onset of dementia with focal neurologic features
- Step-wise decline in cognition

Features unsupportive of vascular dementia include:

- Absence of neurologic signs other than cognitive decline
- Aphasic disturbances without corresponding lesions on imaging
- Patchy or periventricular white matter lesions affecting < 25% of white matter
- Absence of discrete infarctions (ie, visible on T1-weighted MRI)
- Absence of vasculopathic risk factors (eg, hypertension, diabetes mellitus, peripheral arterial disease, coronary artery disease, etc)

Abstracted from Chui et al[14] and Roman et al.[15]

vation is caused by progressive occlusion of arteries. The concept of multi-infarct dementia (MID) arose in the mid-1970s, proposing that discrete cerebral infarctions or strokes were required for the development of dementia.

The emergence of easily available magnetic resonance imaging (MRI) has once again clouded the diagnostic approach to dementia and strokes by revealing changes in cerebral architecture that are not necessarily pathologic or associated with clinical signs. MID is best considered a subtype of vascular dementia (VaD). Binswanger's disease is a term sometimes used synonymously with VaD in the absence of discrete infarcts, but it is primarily a neuropathologic diagnosis without a unitary clinical syndrome. Essentially, any disease associated with cerebral ischemia or hemorrhage can be considered a contributor to vascular dementia. Examples are listed in Table 4.

Therefore, although vascular disease is the second or third most common contributor to dementia, VaD is probably the most overdiagnosed form of dementia. Recently developed criteria have assisted in the research diagnosis of VaD,[6,7] but they offer little validity in comparison to each other and remain cumbersome for routine clinical use.[16] Key diagnostic elements of VaD are shown in Table 5. Degenerative dementing illnesses typically affect older adults, and they do not provide immunity from other age-related illnesses like stroke. Therefore, even when criteria for VaD are met, concurrent vascular and degenerative pathologies are common. Autopsies suggest that Alzheimer-type findings and probable vascular causes of dementia occur together about as often as vascular findings alone.[17]

Cognitive and Behavioral Findings

The accumulation of ischemic brain lesions is typically associated with incremental impairment of memory and behavioral initiation, although a more insidiously progressive course is not unusual. The typical cognitive pattern in vascular dementia includes prominent frontal/executive dysfunction, generally with less language impairment than seen in AD. Focal cortical signs such as visuospatial dysfunction and apraxia occur only when relevant areas of the brain have sustained cerebrovascular lesions.

Physical Findings

A history of acute unilateral motor or sensory dysfunction consistent with stroke can be obtained in about 90% of pathologically verified cases of the multi-infarct form of VaD.[18] Urinary dysfunction and gait disturbances have been suggested as early markers of VaD. Facial masking, rigidity, Babinski's sign, and gait disturbances are common. Early emergence of urinary incontinence can also suggest vascular dementia.

Imaging

Nonspecific findings like periventricular white matter change, as depicted by brain computed tomography (CT) or MRI scans, are insufficient for the diagnosis of VaD. Many of the changes observed on MRI represent the effects of healthy aging, including dilated perivascular spaces. The typical changes include small, focal areas of increased signal, as well as patchy or confluent periventricular white matter hyperintensity on T2-weighted images. An important fact is that a large volume (25% or more) of diffuse signal change may be present on CT or MRI without meaningful impairment of cognition. Cavities present on T1-weighted images are the finding most specific for cerebral infarction.

Despite the lack of a unitary clinical syndrome and the frequent ambiguity of cerebral imaging, the diagnosis of VaD should be strongly considered when multiple vasculopathic risk factors (such as hypertension, coronary disease, previous stroke/transient ischemic attack, etc) are present and extrapyramidal or focal signs are detected on neurologic examination, but AD's cognitive profile is not observed.

Epidemiology

There appear to be no risks specific for the development of VaD within the context of cerebrovascular disease. The absence of consensus criteria for vascular dementia before the 1990s has limited our understanding of the epidemiology of this disease; consequently, much of the literature is based on the construct of MID. The reported frequency of MID in demented populations ranges from 4.5% to 39%, with a best overall estimate of about 10%.[19] The frequency of purely vascular changes in autopsies of demented patients is 10% to 23%, comparable to that of 'mixed dementia' with changes of both MID and AD.[17] Men are affected more often than women, probably reflecting gender influences on stroke risk factors.

Frontotemporal Dementia

In 1892, Pick described the case of a 71-year-old man with progressive cognitive decline, behavioral disturbance, and language impairment. Pathologic changes of argyrophilic cytoplasmic inclusions (Pick's bodies) and marked neuronal dropout in frontal and temporal cortex were later identified in similar cases, and led to the characterization of Pick's disease as one of the classic neurodegenerative disorders. More recently, increasing sophistication in the clinical assessment of dementia and the identification of patients with a clinical syndrome similar to Pick's, but lacking its distinctive pathology, have led to use of the broader term of *frontotemporal dementia* (FTD) to describe these cases. This has led to controversy and ambiguity in classification. For example, DSM-IV and the ICD-9-CM coding scheme do not use FTD as a diagnosis. Other terms such as Pick's disease, dementia of the frontal type, and frontal lobe dementia are used interchangeably in the literature. Consensus diagnostic criteria for FTD have been published[20]; key points for diagnosing FTD are summarized in Table 6.

Cognitive and Behavioral Findings

Frontotemporal dementia most often presents with disturbed behavior rather than decline in cognitive tasks. Poor personal and social judgment are its hallmarks. Perseveration and stereotypy may also be seen. Clinically, disordered initiation, goal-setting, and planning (ie, executive function) are accompanied by

Table 6: Key Points for Diagnosing Frontotemporal Dementia

Diagnostic features of frontotemporal dementia include:

I. A progressive course

II. Either of two major clinical syndromes:

A. Loss of judgment accompanied by one or more of the following:
- disinhibition,
- social misconduct, or
- withdrawal or apathy

or

B. Loss of expressive language or comprehension, or both

III. The changes in point II are proportionately worse than the degree of memory loss or spatial disorientation.

The diagnosis of FTD is *not* supported by:

A. The presence of severe early memory loss or spatial disorientation with less impaired language or executive function

B. The presence of extrapyramidal features on neurologic examination

C. History of another recognized neurologic disorder sufficient to explain the frontotemporal deficits

Abstracted from Knopman,[22] Lund and Manchester Groups[20]

apathetic or disinhibited behavior. Most patients have little awareness of these changes and actively deny or refute any problems (anosognosia). Performance on cognitive screening tests, like the Mini-Mental State Examination, is often normal or minimally impaired. Although any combination of symptoms is possible as the illness progresses, most patients present with either a syndrome of sluggishness with apathy, inertia, and aspontaneity, or a hyperkinetic state of restlessness, distractibility, and disinhibition.[21] The latter presentation often has a hypomanic character. The impaired praxis and visuospatial function characteristic of AD are usually not seen in individuals with frontal lobe dementia until late in the course, if at all. Often, the distinctive 'frontal' pattern of FTD disappears as other areas of cognition worsen.

The classically described Pick's disease is one kind of frontotemporal dementia. It is characterized by motor speech disorders and verbal stereotypies. Language impairments such as abundant unfocused speech (logorrhea), echo-like spontaneous repetition (echolalia), and compulsively uttered repetitive phrases (palilalia) are often seen in conjunction with the behavioral disturbances and may represent focal involvement of language cortices.

Another variant of FTD is known as primary progressive aphasia. Anomia, frequent paraphasic utterances, and reduced speech fluency are common early manifestations. Comprehension is affected less often. Over years, other cognitive functions may decline, but language disturbance remains predominant. Generally, there is less loss of personal or social judgment than typically seen in FTD.

Some cases of FTD present with a typical pattern of poor judgment and behavioral disturbance, but rapidly evolve to include generalized motor dysfunction. A combined upper and lower motor neuron disease pattern such as amyotrophic lateral sclerosis (Lou Gehrig's disease) may be seen. Some individuals develop bulbar palsy with impaired swallowing. Familial forms of FTD that localize to chromosome 17 are also associated with prominent parkinsonism, motor neuron disease, or aphasia. Progressive subcortical gliosis is a rare but neuropathologically well-characterized dementing illness that presents as FTD and may also be linked to chromosome 17. These syndromes may reflect mutations in the tau protein, which localizes to chromosome 17.

Epidemiology

In one large-scale epidemiological study,[23] the prevalence of FTD was estimated at 10.7 per 100,000 in the 50- to 60-year age group and 28 per 100,000 in the 60- to 70-year age group. In practice, the prevalence varies widely with the population. In psychiatric referral populations, FTD may account for up to one sixth of dementia cases, but in general or neurologic practices, the rate is closer to 5% to 10%. The average age of onset is in the mid-50s, which is lower than for AD. A history of dementia was found in 38% of first-degree relatives of FTD probands compared to 15% in nondemented controls.[23]

Creutzfeldt-Jakob and Other Prion Diseases

This group of illnesses is also known as the spongiform encephalopathies. They are associated with infective transmission by a novel, proteinaceous particle known as a prion. Other mammals also harbor variants of these diseases. Cross-species transmission has been identified (eg, mad cow disease). Host genetic factors are also related to the expression of this class of disease, and specific gene markers now allow molecular genetic differentiation of these diseases.

Creutzfeldt-Jakob Disease (CJD)

CJD is the prototypical human disease caused by prions. CJD is a rare, rapidly progressive dementia, first recognized about 1920. Despite the traditional classification of CJD as a transmissible disease, familial forms have now been identified. Gerstmann-Sträussler-Scheinker syndrome (GSSS) is an even rarer but well-recognized autosomal dominant prion syndrome, with prominent ataxia.[24]

Clinical Expression

The classic triad of CJD involves dementia, myoclonus, and a distinctive periodic discharge pattern on electroencephalography. Vague initial symptoms of irritability and unusual somatic sensations occur in about one third of cases. Complex visual dysfunction is a common part of the cognitive loss. One recognized clinical pattern of CJD, known as the Heidenhain variant, is characterized by prominent involvement of higher visual function. It may be confused for AD or variants such as posterior cortical atrophy. Signs of cerebellar dysfunction are also frequent. In addition to the myoclonus, motor signs, such as parkinsonism and motor neuron dysfunction, evolve in many cases.

The rate of progression distinguishes CJD from nearly all other forms of dementia. Patients exhibit overt changes in cognitive and functional ability from month to month, or even more rapidly. Most patients become akinetic and mute within 6 months of diagnosis and die within 1 year. GSSS generally follows a slower course than CJD. Cerebellar findings in GSSS are more pronounced and the dementia is less prominent.

Epidemiology

Most cases occur between the ages of 55 and 75. Mean age of onset is in the early 60s.[25] The annual incidence is about 1 per million overall and 5 to 6 per million in the age range of maximum risk.[26] The very aggressive course leads to a prevalence similar to the incidence. Men and women appear to be at equal risk, and 5% to 10% of cases are familial.

Fatal Familial Insomnia

This bizarre prion-based illness was first recognized in 1986.[27] Insomnia is typically the first symptom. Early complaints of troubled sleep progress over months to a near total inability to sleep, characterized by a severe, persistent, and complete disorganization of the sleep cycle. Cognitive disturbances occur, including deficits in atten-

Table 7: Key Elements for the Diagnosis of Progressive Supranuclear Palsy

Clinical features of PSP include:

I. Progressive disease course including:

   A. Restriction of voluntary vertical gaze, especially downgaze

   B. Postural instability with unexplained falls

II. Supportive findings include:

   A. Impaired cognition with prominent dysexecutive findings

   B. Akinetic-rigid syndrome with neck > limb rigidity

   C. Dysarthria, dysphagia, or pseudobulbar palsy

   D. Minimal levodopa response

III. Findings not supportive:

   A. Unilateral parkinsonism

   B. Early or prominent cerebellar findings

   C. Onset before age 50 or after age 75

Abstracted from Litvan et al[30]

---

tion, memory, and executive function. An apathetic indifference, reduced emotional expression, and prolonged episodes of stupor appear as the illness progresses. Stuporous episodes are frequently associated with motor automatisms, and patients may appear to be acting out dreams. Wide-ranging dysautonomia appears early in the course. It is often followed by motor disturbances, including dysarthria and ataxia.[28] Through 1998, only 13 kindreds have been identified worldwide (3 in North

America). Given the wide geographic distribution of the kindreds, it seems likely that more will be recognized.

Progressive Supranuclear Palsy (PSP)

PSP was first reported by Steele, Richardson, and Olszewski in 1964.[29] Although 7 of the original 9 cases were reported to have cognitive deficits, more attention has been focused on the parkinsonian motor dysfunction and eye-movement disturbance of the syndrome. The characteristic oculomotor finding is impairment of vertical gaze, especially downward. Other eye-movement disorders commonly accompany the vertical gaze paresis. Several sets of criteria have been proposed for the clinical diagnosis of PSP and have been compared for their diagnostic utility.[30] Key diagnostic points are shown in Table 7.

Cognitive and Behavioral Findings

Dementia occurs in 60% to 80% of affected individuals, but is not a necessary part of the syndrome.[31] Generalized cognitive slowing and prominent executive function deficits are typical. The memory deficit is primarily based on difficulty accessing stored material, so recall is better facilitated by cueing or recognition testing than is typical for AD. Object naming and the semantic aspects of language are also not as impaired as in AD (when matched for overall dementia severity). Spatial allocation of attention is also disrupted in PSP,[32] and oculomotor control deficits with resultant visuoperceptual difficulties may cause some of the deficits on neuropsychologic testing.[33] Even after accounting for these motor influences, the cognitive pattern in PSP is unique.

Physical Findings

Postural instability is the most frequent initial symptom, and is often reported as falls. As with DLB, tremor is not a major feature. Rigidity usually affects the neck and trunk rather than the limbs and, when coupled with oculomotor deficits, can lead to disabling difficulties in orienting visual attention. Affected individuals may there-

---

Table 8: Key Elements for Diagnosing Corticobasal Degeneration (CBD)

I. Clinical features suggesting CBD:

    A. Progressive disease course

    B. Unilateral akinetic-rigid syndrome

    C. Apraxia or alien-hand phenomenon (ipsilateral to akinesia/rigidity)

    D. Mild dysexecutive cognitive findings

II. Supportive findings include:

    A. Cortical sensory loss (ipsilateral to akinesia/rigidity)

    B. Action or postural tremor

    C. Orofacial apraxia or aphasia

III. Findings not supportive:

    A. Prominent cognitive or behavioral disturbance

    B. Marked gait abnormality

    C. Dysautonomia

---

fore adopt awkward postures as they attempt to look at items in the environment on command.

Multiple problems with oculomotor control are present in addition to the typical downward-gaze palsy. These include unstable fixation (square-wave jerks), slow saccadic eye movements, and, in more advanced disease, upward and lateral gaze paresis. Speech in PSP includes hypophonia, as in PD, but may also have prominent spastic and ataxic components suggestive of pseudobulbar palsy. The oropharyngeal motor dysfunction is complicated by dysexecutive impulsivity and leads to dysphagia and choking in many patients.

Differential Diagnosis

Litvan et al recently applied an advanced statistical algorithm to identify features differentiating PSP from related disorders.[34] Gait disturbance, limited tremor, and poor response to levodopa best distinguished PSP from idiopathic PD, which is the most common differential. In addition, the eye-movement disorder, a higher degree of gait disturbance, and lack of delusions best differentiated PSP from DLB. Postural instability best differentiated PSP from Pick's disease.

Epidemiology

The age-adjusted prevalence of PSP is 1 to 2 cases per 100,000 population.[35] The annual incidence is therefore estimated at 3 to 4 cases per million population per year. This makes PSP slightly more common than CJD, but about 1% as common as AD or PD. Men are affected slightly more often than women. The age range for onset of PSP is relatively narrow. About 50% of PSP patients develop initial symptoms during their 60s, with remaining cases split equally between their 50s and 70s.[35,36] Median survival is 5 to 6 years.[37]

Corticobasal Degeneration (CBD)

This increasingly recognized cause of parkinsonism with dementia was first recognized by Rebeiz in 1967. Several names have been previously applied, including corticodentatonigral degeneration with achromasia, corticonigral degeneration, and cortical-basal ganglionic degeneration. Key diagnostic points are listed in Table 8.

Cognitive and Behavioral Findings

The most prominent cognitive feature of CBD is apraxia with both ideomotor and ideational components.[38] This is almost always unilateral and associated with a progressive loss of voluntary control of one limb in the absence of objective weakness. The affected limb appears to act independently of the person's other activities. This bizarre finding has been called the *alien limb phenomenon*. Cognitive impairments are otherwise mild in most cases. They typically include a dysexecutive state and impairments in learning new information.[39] Dementia occurs in 25% to 50% of cases, usually quite late in the course.[40-42]

Physical Findings

Unilateral parkinsonian signs of rigidity and bradykinesia are the most common presenting features, occurring in more than 80% of cases.[32] Apractic clumsiness of one hand is often interpreted as an extrapyramidal feature rather than apraxia. As in DLB and PSP, tremor is seen less frequently than rigidity. When tremor occurs, it is often not a typical parkinsonian rest tremor, and often includes concomitant elements of postural and action tremor, sometimes with superimposed dystonia. Cortical sensory loss may present early in the disease, but affects only about one third of patients.[40,42] Rigidity, akinesia, apraxia, and alien limb phenomena may all contribute to dystonic posturing and complete loss of voluntary control of the arm. Either aphasia or a dysfluent aphasia-like language disturbance resulting from orofacial apraxia may be manifest, but these occur in only a minority of cases.[40,41]

Differential Diagnosis

Unilateral cortical sensory loss is the most useful feature distinguishing CBD when it is present. Generally, the diagnosis of CBD should not be made in individuals with prominent dementia in the absence of severe motor findings.[43] This helps to exclude AD and FTD. In contrast to DLB, apraxia is usually more severe than other cognitive or behavioral disturbances in CBD. Unilateral predominance, the absence of vertical gaze palsy, and intact gait in CBD help to differentiate it from PSP.

Epidemiology

CBD is rare, but the exact incidence and prevalence are unknown. Onset typically occurs in the early 60s. There is a slight predominance of men. Average survival is 5 to 10 years, and death typically results from complications of immobility.

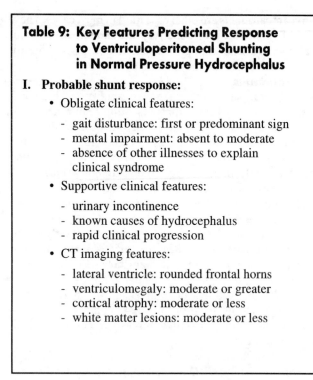

Table 9: Key Features Predicting Response to Ventriculoperitoneal Shunting in Normal Pressure Hydrocephalus

I. Probable shunt response:

- Obligate clinical features:
    - gait disturbance: first or predominant sign
    - mental impairment: absent to moderate
    - absence of other illnesses to explain clinical syndrome
- Supportive clinical features:
    - urinary incontinence
    - known causes of hydrocephalus
    - rapid clinical progression
- CT imaging features:
    - lateral ventricle: rounded frontal horns
    - ventriculomegaly: moderate or greater
    - cortical atrophy: moderate or less
    - white matter lesions: moderate or less

Hydrocephalus

Normal pressure hydrocephalus (NPH) is a rare but potentially reversible form of dementia first described in 1965. It is classically characterized by a triad of gait disorder, urinary incontinence, and cognitive decline, but today is most commonly raised as a part of the differential diagnosis by findings on imaging tests. Each of the 3 clinical elements is relatively common in elderly individuals, and their concurrence in the presence of brain atrophy on cerebral imaging is not sufficient for the diagnosis of NPH.

The basis of the neurologic dysfunction is poor absorption of cerebrospinal fluid (CSF) with subsequent expan-

II. Improbable shunt response*:

- Clinical features:
  - gait disturbance: absent
  - dementia: prominent or early
  - predominance of cortical signs (aphasia, apraxia, agnosia)
  - presence of another disease consistent with syndrome (eg, vascular dementia)
- CT imaging features:
  - lateral ventricle/ventriculomegaly: slight dilatation
  - cortical atrophy: marked
  - white matter lesions: severe

* Any one of these findings make shunt response unlikely.

Adapted from Vanneste et al.[44]

sion of the lateral ventricles. Ventricular enlargement stretches or distorts frontal lobe axons involved in cognition as well as lower extremity and urinary bladder control, with resultant dysfunction in these systems. Definitive treatment is usually ventriculoperitoneal shunting. A combination of clinical and imaging criteria can be used to predict response to shunting[44] (Table 9).

Clinical Expression

In most patients, the gait disorder appears first, followed by the cognitive changes. The gait dysfunction is characterized by short steps and poor turning ability, but usually lacks the shuffling character associated with parkinsonian syndromes. Instead, the gait has been described as *magnetic*, and patients may report they feel as though their feet are stuck to the floor. Rigidity, spasticity, and hyperreflexia of the legs may also evolve. Cognitive symptoms are typically mild and include psychomotor slowing, with impaired concentration and mild memory difficulties. Focal cortical symptoms (such as the aphasia, apraxia, and agnosia characteristic of AD) are exceptionally rare, as is psychosis. Urinary incontinence is variably expressed and may not occur. Since prostatism in men and stress incontinence in women are common in the age groups at risk for NPH, the predictive value of incontinence is low.

Gait disturbance is the most likely symptom to improve with CSF diversion. The probability of cognitive improvement after shunting is generally low, but best when the dementia is of short duration. The best outcomes are seen in individuals with mild to moderate gait disturbance and dementia along with no cortical atrophy and no severe white matter changes on imaging. Conversely, severe dementia, significant cortical atrophy, or severe white matter disease indicate poor symptomatic resolution with shunting.

Although no test is ideal, a positive CSF-tap test remains the best clinical predictor of treatment success with ventriculoperitoneal shunting. It is, however, complicated by a high false-negative rate. Some clinicians use serial lumbar punctures to manage this illness or to assess likelihood of successful shunting. Radioisotope cisternography is commonly used to assist in diagnosis, but it has been reported as unreliable for predicting surgical outcome.[44]

Paraneoplastic Limbic Encephalitis

A subacute cognitive or behavioral disorder can complicate some forms of cancer, particularly small cell lung tumors. Neuronal loss results from autoimmune mechanisms in which the affected neurons are innocent bystanders that share antigenic properties with the neoplastic cells. In many cases, the neuropsychiatric manifestations predate discovery of the tumor by months or, rarely, years. Memory dysfunction, particularly acquisition of new information, is typical. The historical use of the term *limbic encephalitis* represents the predominance of affective and emotional findings in many patients. These include anxiety, depression, emotional lability, irritability, and personality change. Other neurologic changes may also be present, including somnolence, inattentiveness, motor signs, and dysautonomia.

Dementia in Other Neurologic Disease

Any illness that disrupts the intricate architecture of cerebral neuronal connections can disrupt cognition. A number of neurodegenerative diseases usually do not have dementia as their initial manifestation, but can develop prominent cognitive or behavioral dysfunction as they progress. These will be reviewed briefly.

Idiopathic Parkinson's Disease (PD)

Although James Parkinson initially reported that intellect was spared during the course of *paralysis agitans*, cognitive changes can be detected in many patients with idiopathic PD. The overall prevalence of dementia in PD is controversial, but is probably about one third. Dementia is rare in PD patients below the age of 60, but by age 85, more than 65% of PD patients in one study had developed significant cognitive decline.[45] Patients with a family history of dementia appear to have a higher risk for the development of dementia with PD.

Visuospatial dysfunction and executive function abnormalities are common in PD. These cognitive changes occur even in tests that control for the motor disability. Psychiatric changes also occur, particularly depression (which can occur in up to 90% of patients with PD). Delusions and hallucinations also occur, especially in advanced PD. They are often exacerbated by treatment with dopaminergic agents.

Huntington's Disease

Huntington's disease (HD) is an autosomal, dominantly inherited neurologic illness with clinical characteristics of abnormal movements and neuropsychiatric disturbances, including delusions, depression, and mania. Cognitive symptoms include problems with attention and concentration, memory, and executive function. Aphasic characteristics are uncommon, though dysarthria may result from the motor disabilities. In contrast to other dementia forms such as AD, which can cause preferential loss of fact-based memory, HD has a major effect on procedural (or skill-based) memory.[46]

The classic motor finding in HD is chorea or, more properly, choreoathetosis. This consists of involuntary twitching movements of the distal extremities (chorea) which progress to more writhing (athetoid) movements proximally. Marked atrophy of the caudate nuclei is usually visible on cerebral imaging.

Epidemiology

Onset is typically in the 30s or early 40s, although some cases have later onset and long duration of illness. Few new cases appear after age 70. The prevalence is about 5 to 10 per 100,000 in whites of European origin, and lower among those of African or Asian ancestry. A trinucleotide repeat form of genetic defect localizes to the short arm of chromosome 4. Reliable genetic testing is available, although the ethical implications are complex for presymptomatic diagnosis of this illness.

Other Illnesses

Specific clinical or pathologic features can identify other rare dementias, but atypical forms of dementia can be extremely difficult to differentiate during life. Some cases of progressive dementia lack any distinctive histopathology and have been called *simple atrophy*. About 1% to 2% of cases of sporadic amyotrophic lateral sclerosis are also associated with dementia, typically with a symptom pattern like FTD. The familial cerebellar degenerations also may include cognitive changes, typically with dysexecutive findings.

Alcohol

Alcohol abuse is often considered a cause of dementia, but it is unclear that a primary alcohol-related dementia exists, since no distinctive pattern of clinical symptoms or neuropathology has been identified. Several syndromes that have a strong association with alcohol abuse do lead to cognitive deficits, but probably through nutritional deficiencies. They include Korsokoff's syndrome, which is always linked to an episode of Wernicke's encephalitis in the context of acute thiamine deficiency. Korsokoff's syndrome is an anterograde amnesia syndrome with a disabling limitation of memory span. A fixed retrograde memory loss may occur as well. Patients with Korsokoff's syndrome often cannot remember information for as long as 1 minute and frequently confabulate. Pellagra, the clinical syndrome of nicotinic acid deficiency, also leads to cognitive impairments in alcohol abusers. Marchiafava-Bignami syndrome is a dementing syndrome pathologically characterized by degeneration or necrosis of the corpus callosum. It is associated with heavy alcohol use. The clinical features include a dysexecutive syndrome and apraxia, leading to possible confusion with CBD.

HIV

Dementia occurs in up to one third of individuals with HIV infection, but is the sole presenting symptom in less than 5% of cases. Psychomotor slowing and focal neurologic signs often characterize HIV-related dementias. HIV testing is warranted in those with known risk behaviors and in patients whose routine clinical, imaging, and laboratory tests fail to identify likely causes of dementia. Progressive multifocal leukoencephalopathy is another dementing syndrome associated with immunocompromise. Like HIV-related dementia, systemic signs usually predate cognitive decline.

Syphilis

General paresis is the historical term used to describe the very late effect of syphilitic infections of the brain. Like the closely related spinal cord syndrome known as tabes dorsalis, syphilitic dementia occurs 15 to 30 years after acute exposure. In the preantibiotic era, this was a common cause of early-onset dementia, but now, other than certain high-risk groups (eg, HIV patients), late syphilis is exceptionally rare. Dementia caused by syphilis is typically associated with prominent behavioral disturbances, including delusions, emotional lability, hallucinations, and mania. When serum markers of syphilis are identified, especially treponemal-specific tests (eg, FTA-ABS or MHATP), lumbar puncture is indicated. A positive spinal fluid serology is, however, insufficient to diagnose general paresis, because these markers can remain positive throughout life. Generally, a CSF white blood cell count of > 5/mm^3 is necessary to consider a full treatment course of IV antibiotics for neurosyphilis. Dementia should not be expected to resolve, but slowing of progression may be possible.

Thyroid Dysfunction

Hypothyroidism leads to slowness, inattention, apathy, lethargy, and depression. More severe hypothyroidism can produce frank dementia. Psychotic features occur in 3% to 5% of patients with severe hypothyroidism.[47] Only rarely do the cognitive features emerge without the classical systemic features of hypothyroidism. These include fatigue, lethargy, constipation, cold intolerance, menorrhagia, reduced appetite, weight gain, dry skin, dryness and thinning of the hair, and deepening of the voice.

Hyperthyroidism results in nervousness, irritability, restlessness, hyperkinesia, emotional lability, and inability to concentrate. Confusion and poor performance on cognitive testing may result from reduced ability to focus or concentrate. Paradoxically, depression may be present, but anxiety or mania are more common.[48] As with hypothyroidism, systemic evidence of the disorder is almost always evident when neuropsychiatric manifestations evolve. Neurologic signs, particularly tremor, are frequent.

Vasculitis

Cerebral vasculitides are a group of disorders of widely disparate causes that may present with cognitive disorders. As with HIV, the systemic illness is apparent before signs of cognitive or behavioral disorder in most individuals. Primary angiitis of the central nervous system (CNS) is, however, an extremely rare vasculitic syndrome that presents with dementia. About 30% of patients with this disorder have cognitive impairment at first presentation.[49] The disorder is characterized by progressive cognitive decline over months in the absence of systemic signs. The symptom pattern depends on the areas of brain affected by the patchy inflammation, but most commonly includes prominent executive function and attention deficits. Primary CNS angiitis may present throughout adult life, without a strong weighting toward the elderly. Diagnosis depends on clinical suspicion, cerebral angiography, and meningeal/brain biopsy.

Vitamin B$_{12}$ Deficiency

Deficiency of this vitamin can produce disturbances of mental function, but usually in the context of other neurologic features such as peripheral neuropathy and subacute combined degeneration of the posterior and lateral columns of the spinal cord. Nonetheless, cognitive dysfunction can occur years before hematologic or spinal cord symptoms appear. Numbness and tingling (paraesthesia) in the limbs is the most frequent neurologic symptom. Forgetfulness and irritability are the most common neuropsychiatric features, although psychosis and severe dementia have been seen with protracted Vitamin B$_{12}$ deficiency. Among patients with neuropsychiatric abnormalities secondary to B_{12} deficiency, as many as 28% have no anemia or macrocytosis.[50] Complete resolution of dementia with treatment is unusual.

References

1. Goldman WP, Morris JC: Evidence that age-associated memory impairment is not a normal variant of aging. *Alzheimer Dis Assoc Disord* 2001;15:72-79.

2. Crook TH, Bartus R, Ferris SH, et al: Age-associated memory impairment: proposed diagnostic criteria and measures of clinical change: report of a National Institutes of Mental Health work group. *Dev Neuropsychol* 1986;2:261-276.

3. Levy R: Aging-associated cognitive decline. Working Party of the International Psychogeriatric Association in collaboration with the World Health Organization. *Int Psychogeriatr* 1994;6:63-68.

4. Larrabee GJ, Crook TH: Estimated prevalence of age-associated memory impairment derived from standardized tests of memory function. *Int Psychogeriatr* 1994;6:95-104.

5. Petersen RC, Stevens JC, Ganguli M, et al: Practice parameter: early detection of dementia: mild cognitive impairment (an evidence-based review). Report of the Quality Standards Subcommittee of the American Academy of Neurology. *Neurology* 2001;56: 1133-1142.

6. Petersen RC, Doody R, Kurz A, et al: Current concepts in mild cognitive impairment. *Arch Neurol* 2001;58:1985-1992.

7. Ritchie K, Artero S, Touchon J, et al: Classification criteria for mild cognitive impairment: a population-based validation study. *Neurology* 2001;56:37-42.

8. Wentzel C, Rockwood K, MacKnight C, et al: Progression of impairment in patients with vascular cognitive impairment without dementia. *Neurology* 2001;57:714-716.

9. Alexopolous GS, Meyers BS, Young RC, et al: The course of geriatric depression with 'reversible dementia': a controlled study. *Am J Psychiatry* 1993;150:1693-1699.

10. Cummings JL, Benson DF: *Dementia: A Clinical Approach*, 2nd ed. Boston, Butterworth-Heinemann, 1992.

11. Luis CA, Barker WW, Gajaraj K, et al: Sensitivity and specificity of three clinical criteria for dementia with Lewy bodies in an autopsy-verified sample. *Int J Geriatric Psychiatry* 1999;14:526-533.

12. McKeith IG, Galasko D, Kosaka K, et al: Consensus guidelines for the clinical and pathological diagnosis of dementia with Lewy bodies (DLB): report of the consortium on DLB international workshop. *Neurology* 1996;47:1113-1124.

13. Kalra S, Bergeron C, Lang AE: Lewy body disease and dementia: a review. *Arch Intern Med* 1996;156:487-493.

14. Chui HC, Victoroff JI, Margolin D, et al: Criteria for ischemic vascular dementia proposed by the State of California Alzheimer's Disease Diagnostic and Treatment Centers. *Neurology* 1992; 42:473-480.

15. Roman GC, Tatemichi TK, Erkinjuntti T, et al: Vascular dementia: diagnostic criteria for research studies: report of the NINDS-AIREN International Workshop. *Neurology* 1993;43:250-260.

16. Wetterling T, Kanitz R, Borgis K: Comparison of different diagnostic criteria for vascular dementia (ADDTC, DSM-IV, ICD-10, NINDS-AIREN). *Stroke* 1996;27:30-36.

17. Katzman R, Lasker B, Bernstein N: Advances in the diagnosis of dementia: accuracy of diagnosis and consequence of misdiagnosis of disorders causing dementia. In: Terry RD, ed. *Aging and the Brain*. New York, Raven Press, 1988, pp 17-62.

18. Erkinjuntti T, Haltia M, Palo J, et al: Accuracy of the clinical diagnosis of vascular dementia: a prospective clinical and postmortem neuropathological study. *J Neurol Neurosurg Psychiatry* 1988;51:1037-1044.

19. Kase CS: Epidemiology of multi-infarct dementia. *Alzheimer Dis Assoc Disord* 1991;5:71-76.

20. Lund and Manchester Groups: Clinical and neuropathological criteria for frontotemporal dementia. *J Neurol Neurosurg Psychiatry* 1994;57:416-418.

21. Neary D, Snowden JS, Northen B, et al: Dementia of frontal lobe type. *J Neurol Neurosurg Psychiatry* 1988;51:353-361.

22. Knopman D: Fronto-temporal dementia. *Neurobase* (electronic reference). San Diego, Arbor Publishing, 1998.

23. Stevens M, van Duijn CM, Kamphorst W, et al: Familial aggregation in frontotemporal dementia. *Neurology* 1998;50:1541-1545.

24. Kitamoto T, Yamaguchi K, Dohura K, et al: A prion protein missense variant is integrated in kuru plaque cores in patients with Gerstmann-Straussler syndrome. *Neurology* 1991;41:306-310.

25. Brown P, Cathala F, Castaigne P, et al: Creutzfeldt-Jakob disease: clinical analysis of a consecutive series of 230 neuropathologically verified cases. *Ann Neurol* 1986;20:597-602.

26. Holman RC, Khan AS, Kent J, et al: Epidemiology of Creutzfeldt-Jakob disease in the United States, 1979-1990: analysis of national mortality data. *Neuroepidemiology* 1995;14:174-181.

27. Lugaresi E, Medori R, Montagna P, et al: Fatal familial insomnia and dysautonomia with selective degeneration of thalamic nuclei. *N Engl J Med* 1986;315:997-1003.

28. Gallassi R, Morreale A, Montagna P, et al: Fatal familial insomnia: behavioral and cognitive features. *Neurology* 1996;46:935-939.

29. Steele JC, Richardson JC, Olszewski J: Progressive supranuclear palsy. *Arch Neurol* 1964;10:333-359.

30. Litvan I, Agid Y, Jankovic J, et al: Accuracy of the clinical criteria for the diagnosis of progressive supranuclear palsy (Steele-Richardson-Olszewski syndrome). *Neurology* 1996;46:922-930.

31. Maher ER, Smith EM, Lees AJ: Cognitive deficits in the Steele-Richardson-Olszewski syndrome (progressive supranuclear palsy). *J Neurol Neurosurg Psychiatry* 1985;48:1234-1239.

32. Grafman J, Litvan I, Stark M: Neuropsychological features of progressive supranuclear palsy. *Brain Cogn* 1995;28:311-320.

33. Podoll K, Schwartz M, Noth J: Language function in progressive supranuclear palsy. *Brain* 1991;114:1457-1472.

34. Litvan I, Campbell G, Mangone CA, et al: Which clinical features differentiate progressive supranuclear palsy (Steele-Richardson-Olszewski syndrome) from related disorders: a clinicopathologic study. *Brain* 1997;120:65-74.

35. Golbe LI, Davis PH, Schoenberg BS, et al: Prevalence and natural history of progressive supranuclear palsy. *Neurology* 1988;38:1031-1034.

36. Maher ER, Lees AJ: The clinical features and natural history of the Steele-Richardson-Olszewski syndrome (progressive supranuclear palsy). *Neurology* 1986;36:1005-1008.

37. Litvan I, Mangone CA, McKee A, et al: Progressive supranuclear palsy (Steele-Richardson-Olszewski syndrome) and clinical predictors of survival: a clinicopathologic study. *J Neurol Neurosurg Psychiatry* 1996;61:615-620.

38. Heilman KM: The apraxia of CBGD. *Mov Disord* 1996;11:348.

39. Pillon B, Blin J, Vidailhet M, et al: The neuropsychological pattern of corticobasal degeneration: comparison with progressive supranuclear palsy and Alzheimer's disease. *Neurology* 1995;45:1477-1483.

40. Riley DE, Lang AE, Lewis A, et al: Cortical-basal ganglionic degeneration. *Neurology* 1990;40:1203-1212.

41. Rinne JO, Lee MS, Thompson PD, et al: Corticobasal degeneration: a clinical study of 36 cases. *Brain* 1994;117:1183-1196.

42. Kompolito K, Goetz C, Boeve BF, et al: Clinical presentation and pharmacological response in corticobasal degeneration. *Arch Neurol* 1998;55:957-961.

43. Lang AE, Bergeron C, Pollanen MS, et al: Parietal Pick's disease mimicking cortical-basal ganglionic degeneration. *Neurology* 1994;44:1436-1440.

44. Vanneste J, Augustijn P, Tan WF, et al: Shunting normal pressure hydrocephalus: the predictive value of combined clinical and CT data. *J Neurol Neurosurg Psychiatry* 1993;56:251-256.

45. Mayeux R, Chen J, Mirabello E, et al: An estimate of the incidence of dementia in idiopathic Parkinson's disease. *Neurology* 1990;40:1513-1517.

46. Knopman D, Nissen MJ: Procedural learning is impaired in Huntington's disease: evidence from the serial reaction time task. *Neuropsychologia* 1991;29:245-254.

47. Swanson JR, Kelly JJ, McConahey WM: Neurologic aspects of thyroid dysfunction. *Mayo Clin Proc* 1981;56:504-512.

48. Jadresic DP: Psychiatric aspects of hyperthyroidism. *J Psychosom Res* 1990;34:603-615.

49. Abu Shakra M, Khraishi M, Grosman H, et al: Primary angiitis of the CNS diagnosed by angiography. *Q J Med* 1994;87:351-358.

50. Lindenbaum J, Healton EB, Savage DG, et al: Neuropsychiatric disorders caused by cobalamin deficiency in the absence of anemia or macrocytosis. *N Engl J Med* 1988;318:1720-1728.

Chapter 5

Clinical Approach to Dementia Diagnosis

The clinical approach to diagnosis in dementia is not, as some might suggest, a mysterious art best reserved for wizards in dark robes and pointed hats. Nor need it be restricted to white-coated professors in academic ivory towers. Primary care providers will remain at the forefront of dementia diagnosis and care because of the burgeoning number of people at risk for dementia and because of the continuing evolution of health-care economics.

AD's clinical syndrome is well described by the National Institute of Neurological and Communicative Disorders and the Alzheimer's Disease and Related Disorders Association (NINCDS-ADRDA) criteria.[1] Key elements of these criteria are depicted in Table 1. When the clinical elements of probable AD are present, the likelihood of a pathologic diagnosis of AD is 80% to 90%. Simply put, AD should no longer be considered a diagnosis of exclusion.

Fortunately, the general principles of clinical diagnosis—history, examination, and laboratory evaluation—can be applied effectively in diagnosing dementia and distinguishing between its major causes. Guidance is also available for the provider in the form of practice guidelines from several organizations, including the Federal Agency for Health Care Policy and Research,[2] the American Academy of Neurology,[3,4] the American Psychiatric Association,[5] and a consensus conference of The American Association of Geriatric Psychiatry, the Alzheimer's

Association, and the American Geriatrics Society.[6] The approach recommended by the AHCPR guidelines is depicted in Figure 1. Although no longer considered a clinical standard, this approach remains useful for guiding the thought process in evaluating possible dementia. This chapter reviews the practical aspects of clinical diagnosis in dementia.

Using History to Identify Patients at Risk

In most patients, the symptoms of AD follow a predictable clinical progression, which directly reflects the evolution of the neuropathologic burden over time. The early symptoms are subtle and frequently present for years before coming to medical attention. Patients with early dementia are more likely to seek care for other health problems. The AHCPR guidelines, therefore, suggest several findings that should prompt a clinician to evaluate for the presence of dementia, even when cognitive or behavioral changes are not the presenting complaint (Table 2). Questions to elicit these aspects of functional ability can be asked in a nonthreatening manner while obtaining the social history.

By definition, persons with dementia forget things. Consequently, they are poor informants. They may not be able to remember or relate problems clearly, even when coached by concerned family members. Therefore, clinicians should seek corroborating evidence from family members if inconsistencies or excessive vagueness characterize the patient's responses to questioning. Historical information gathered from family members should also include a description of the pattern of onset, initial problems, duration, course, other symptoms, and associated physical findings. Table 3 lists elements of the history vital to differential diagnosis and severity assessment.

The onset of the degenerative forms of dementia is usually insidious. The gradual onset may be so subtle that friends and family miss it. In these cases, family members will often cite a signal event, such as hospitalization or a psychologic

Table 1: Key Elements of the NINCDS-ADRDA Criteria for the Diagnosis of Alzheimer's Disease (AD)

Diagnosis of probable AD requires:

- Presence of a dementia syndrome
- Deficits in 2 or more areas of cognition
- Progressive worsening of memory and other cognitive function
- Onset between ages 40 and 90 (usually after age 65)
- Absence of systemic diseases that could be causing the syndrome

Supportive findings for probable AD include:

- Progressive aphasia, apraxia, agnosia (including visuospatial dysfunction)
- Impaired activities of daily living and behavior change
- Positive family history
- Unrevealing or nonspecific spinal fluid, EEG, and CT scan findings

Features consistent with the diagnosis of probable AD include:

- Plateau in the course of progression of the illness
- Associated psychiatric and vegetative symptoms (eg, depression, insomnia, delusions, hallucinations), behavioral control problems, sleep disruption, and weight loss

- Other neurologic abnormalities in advanced disease (eg, increased muscle tone, myoclonus, or gait disorder)
- Seizures in advanced disease
- CT normal for age

Probable Alzheimer's disease is unlikely with:

- Sudden, apoplectic onset
- Focal neurologic findings early in the course
- Seizures or gait disturbances early in the course

Clinical diagnosis of *possible* AD:

- May be made on the basis of the dementia syndrome when:
    - other neurologic, psychiatric, or systemic disorders sufficient to cause dementia are absent
    - there are atypical features in the onset, presentation, or clinical course
- May be made in the presence of a second disorder that can lead to dementia, but which is not likely to be the sole cause of the dementia

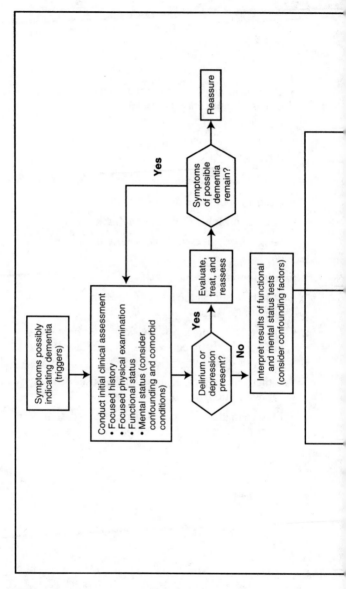

Symptoms possibly indicating dementia (triggers)

Conduct initial clinical assessment
- Focused history
- Focused physical examination
- Functional status
- Mental status (consider confounding and comorbid conditions)

Delirium or depression present?

Yes → Evaluate, treat, and reassess → Symptoms of possible dementia remain? → Yes (back to initial clinical assessment)

Symptoms of possible dementia remain? → Reassure

No → Interpret results of functional and mental status tests (consider confounding factors)

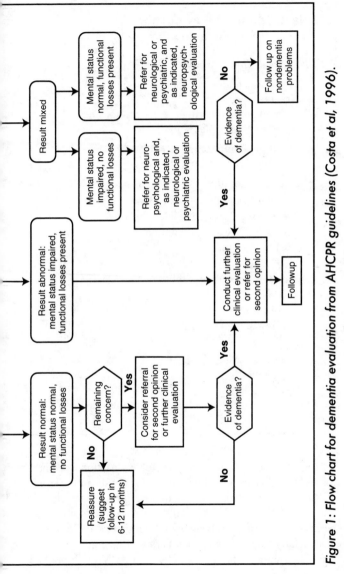

Figure 1: Flow chart for dementia evaluation from AHCPR guidelines (Costa et al, 1996).

Table 2. Triggers for Evaluation of Cognitive Impairment

Difficulties in These Areas:

- Learning and retaining information
  - repetitiveness
  - trouble remembering conversations, etc
  - frequently misplaces items

- Handling complex tasks
  - eg, meal preparation, finances

- Reasoning ability
  - planning and problem solving
  - following rules of social conduct

- Spatial ability and orientation
  - driving
  - household organization
  - finding way around familiar settings

- Language
  - word finding
  - following conversation

- Behavior
  - passive or less responsive
  - irritable
  - suspicious
  - misinterprets visual or auditory stimuli

loss, as the *cause* of dementia. Careful exploration for subtle losses in ability or transitions of responsibility in these patients will often reveal pre-existing or compensated losses that were unmasked by the acute event. Families may also be poor at identifying changes in function that indicate disease. Many times, family members will attribute a loss of functional ability to motivational factors (ie, "My wife cooked for all those years, and I can see how she might not want to anymore"), or to the aging process ("Dad doesn't balance the checkbook as easily as before, but he is nearly 80 now"). Therefore, clinicians should ask specifically about functional changes, such as difficulties with complex meal preparation, finances, or household chores, even though family members may misinterpret the cause of those changes. A family questionnaire developed by the National Chronic Care Consortium and the Alzheimer's Association can be used to characterize deficits in memory and function (Table 4).

If deficits in function or cognition emerge in the history, clinicians must also consider alcohol and over-the-counter, prescriptive or illicit drug use as potential contributors. Drug effects are the most common source of reversible cognitive deficits in older adults.[7] Unintended polypharmacy from multiple providers is a major culprit in this problem. Anticholinergic drugs for GI or GU complaints are common offenders, as are anxiolytics, sedative/hypnotics (including over-the-counter products), and low-potency opioid analgesics such as propoxyphene. Combination preparations for nighttime pain (eg, acetaminophen plus diphenhydramine) or cough-and-cold symptoms can be hidden sources of anticholinergic activity leading to cognitive impairment.

Medication compliance becomes questionable in patients with dementia who manage their medicines, and becomes another potential indicator of meaningful cognitive impairment. Typical medical encounters do not verify medication compliance except through patient report. Almost by definition, patients with dementia become unreliable informants. They tend to provide answers that are socially conforming (eg, "Why, yes, of course I'm taking my medicines, doctor") or that are based on habit rather than on actual recent performance ("I always take everything just the way you prescribe it"). A reasonable screen for cognition can therefore be accomplished with a question such as, "Please tell me how you are taking your medicines." All intact patients should be able to outline the broad schedule

Table 3: Key Features of the Medical History of Dementia

- Pattern of onset?
  - abrupt
  - associated with acute illness or surgery
  - insidious
  - triggered (ie, after retirement or loss of spouse)

- Initial problems?
  - apathy or depression
  - forgetfulness
  - irritability
  - psychosis
  - unusual behavior
  - visual disturbance
  - language disturbance
  - apraxia

- Duration?
  - weeks
  - months
  - years

of their medications, or at least refer to a written list. Those who cannot describe their pattern of taking their pills warrant closer evaluation for possible dementia.

Loss of control in previously controlled illnesses—often hypertension or diabetes—may result from inadvertent noncompliance associated with dementia. Prescriptions for new *additional* agents to treat the same disease state can then lead to 'within-disease polypharmacy.' Therefore, patients with increasing numbers of prescribed medications within-disease should have their compliance verified by pill counts or other tracking mechanisms such as the prescription fulfillment history. For example, is the patient obtaining his or her 30-day or 90-day supply of medication at the

- Course?
  - fluctuating
  - progressive
  - stable

- Other symptoms?
  - change in sleep habits
  - change in urinary habits
  - gait disturbance
  - visual complaints
  - weakness or incoordination

- Impact on function?
  - cooking
  - household chores
  - work performance
  - hobbies
  - interpersonal relationships

appropriate intervals? Forgetting to take pills or failure to obtain refills will lead to a reduced rate of prescription filling. More rarely, patients forget they have taken their dose and will repeat them within the same day. This often has more urgent implications and may be detected by acute symptoms such as syncope or confusion.

A family history of AD is important because it is associated with an increased risk for developing the illness. AD in a first-degree relative (ie, parent or sibling) increases the relative risk for the patient 2- to 5-fold. Clinicians should ask about memory loss rather than AD or dementia, because many other terms for cognitive decline have been used in the past. Family history for stroke is pertinent in the consideration of

Table 4: Family Questionnaire for Early Identification of Dementia

Some older adults develop problems with memory and the ability to think clearly. Even when these occur, they often are not brought to the attention of the physician. Family members or friends of an older person may be aware of problems that should prompt further evaluation by the physician. Please answer the following questionnaire. This information will help us provide better care for your family member.

In your opinion, does _____ have problems with any of the following? Please circle the answer.

1. Repeats or asks the same thing over and over?

   not at all   mild   severe

2. Problems remembering appointments, family occasions, holidays?

   not at all   mild   severe

3. Problems writing checks, paying bills, balancing the checkbook?

   not at all   mild   severe

4. Problems deciding what groceries or clothes to buy?

   not at all   mild   severe

5. Problems taking medications according to instructions?

   not at all   mild   severe

Relationship to patient_____

Scoring:

not at all = 0   mild (a little) = 1   severe (a lot) = 2

Total Score:

vascular dementia. Patients should also be asked about parkinsonism because the clinical differentiation of the many parkinsonian syndromes now recognized is a relatively recent phenomenon. Inaccurate or incomplete characterization of these syndromes remains common.

Screening for Abstract Thought

Abstract thinking is particularly vulnerable early in AD and, therefore, is worth evaluating in older patients who have not been seen previously, or whenever concerns about functional ability arise. This aspect of cognition may be assessed with a simple question that can be disguised as history-taking rather than examination. That question is, "Can you tell me how you like to spend your free time?" This question can be raised as part of the social history to disguise its role in mental state assessment. Responding meaningfully to this question requires recall of broad categories of activity and the formulation of lists. These conceptual (or semantic) abilities are lost early in the course of AD.[8] AD patients are likely to give nonspecific responses like, 'The usual . . .' or perhaps a recitation of daily chores. More appropriate answers generally involve categories such as reading, gardening, or watching television. The clinician should ask the patient to expand upon one of these, eg, by inquiring what kinds of things she likes to read. Again, the patient should be able to provide a list of several examples. Failure to give concrete responses suggests a problem in semantic memory. This gives the clinician the opportunity to express concern about the patient's memory and proceed to more detailed cognitive testing.

A statement like, "It seems to me as though you're having a hard time remembering some of the things you do during the day. I'd like to reassure myself by checking a few things in your memory," allows a relatively nonthreatening transition to cognitive testing. It places the provider in the position of reassurance, eg, "Let me be sure everything is OK," rather than acting from superior knowledge, eg, "I'm

Table 5: Rapid Cognitive Screening Examination for Alzheimer's Disease

Most healthy adults should complete the screening in 5 minutes or less.

I. Assess abstract thinking — "Tell me how you like to spend your spare time.":

    A. If response is suitably abstract and well-formed, *and* there are no cognitive or behavioral complaints, further evaluation can be deferred.

    B. If response is concrete, excessively vague, or details can't be expanded upon, continue on to Part II.

II. Assess focal cortical function:

    A. Learning — "I'd like you to repeat and remember these 3 words: tulip, umbrella, fear."

    B. Working memory/calculation — "If I gave you a penny, a nickel, a dime, and a quarter, how much money would that be?"

    C. Naming — "Please tell me if you remember the name for: (point to jacket, lapel, sleeve, pocket, cuff)."

    D. Temporoparietal tests

       1. "With your right hand, show me how you'd use a hammer to hit a nail."

going to find out what you don't know." The cognitive evaluation can then be directed toward meeting the established criteria for AD or, less often, other causes of dementia.

Screening Focal Cognitive Abilities

Further testing is indicated if screening for abstract thought demonstrates potential problems, or if memory complaints

2. "With your left hand, show me how you'd use a key to open a lock."
3. "Use both hands and show me how you'd slice a loaf of bread."
4. "Touch your left ear with your right hand."
5. "Use your left hand to point to my left hand."
6. "Before pointing to the ceiling, point to the door."

E. Visual constructions

1. "Draw the face of a clock, put the numbers on, and set the time to 8:20."
2. "Copy this drawing."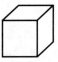

F. Memory — "Please tell me the 3 words I asked you to remember a few minutes ago."

1. spontaneous recall
2. semantic cueing
3. recognition lists

III. Interpretation:

A. If the patient performs well on Part II, reassess in 6-12 months;

B. If the patient performs poorly on 2 or more sections of Part II, more detailed evaluation is required.

or evidence for functional decline are obtained during the medical history. A survey of major cognitive abilities will help to establish the patterns of preserved and impaired abilities. This will assist in understanding which regions of the brain are most affected, and contribute to differential diagnosis. Ideally, a standardized test like the Mini-Mental State Examination (MMSE) should be used.[6] Although this test is simple to administer and well validated, many clinicians consider it too cumbersome or time-consuming for screening purposes. As an alternative, the initial screening cognitive evaluation can focus on identifying the typical patterns and criteria for AD. One example of such an examination is summarized below and outlined in Table 5. A healthy adult should complete these assessments in about 5 minutes. Patients who take longer, even if the answers are correct, should arouse suspicion of impairment.

Learning. The patient should be asked to repeat and remember 3 unrelated words, such as *tulip*, *umbrella*, and *fear*. Word lists that are semantically related, such as *red*, *blue*, and *green*, or *butter*, *eggs*, and *coffee*, are less useful because remembering their theme can make recall easier. The 3 words, also called memory probes, can be repeated as often as necessary to ensure that the patient can repeat all 3 without prompting. Normal performance is to learn and repeat all 3 words with the first exposure. Sometimes a patient with a hearing deficit may misperceive one or more words, eg, 'beer' for 'fear.' When this happens, recall can be assessed for the way the patient repeated the word.

Working memory. After repeating the 3 words, the patient is asked to perform a test of working memory. In addition to testing the patient's ability to work with multiple items simultaneously (an executive function), this occupies the memory system to prevent rehearsal of the 3 memory probes. One useful working memory task asks the patient to add a penny, a dime, a nickel, and a quarter and report how much money the coins represent. It is important that the names of the coins be used, because the working memory system is engaged throughout the subtly complicated process of translating the names to numerical values, performing stepwise addition, and reporting the answer in a unit different than what was provided. Nondemented patients are not overly threatened by this task because it involves familiar items and the everyday activity of adding pocket change.

The task is sufficiently familiar that a pencil and paper are not required for normal performance. The patient who asks for writing tools, or who dismisses the task as something he or she would need to write down should raise suspicion that working memory is impaired. The pocket change addition task is useful as a screening tool because it can assess arithmetic calculation simultaneously with working memory. The patient who answers "36 cents" can add numbers, but has failed to include all 4 coins in working memory. AD patients often struggle laboriously through the process only to answer nonsensically, eg, "62 cents."

Other tests of working memory or related aspects of attention and executive function can be used if pocket change addition is inappropriate (eg, the person is unfamiliar with the common names of US coins). Alternatives include asking the patient to state the months of the year or days of the week in reverse order. These do not, however, incorporate the complexities of translation and addition of the 4 coins.

Naming. A correlate of word-finding difficulty in the spontaneous speech of the AD patient is a reduced ability to name objects or their parts on command. This can be tested with everyday objects available to the examiner, such as a jacket, shoe, or watch. Parts of objects are more difficult to name than whole objects. Therefore, in addition to the jacket as a whole, the patient should be asked to name the collar, lapel, sleeve, pocket, and cuff. Parts of a wristwatch that can be used as naming probes include the band, crystal or face, and crown or stem. In the screening process, naming should be tested in the visual modality. Hints about function should be avoided. Also, responses are considered correct only if the patient provides a reasonable name for the item. Descriptions of appearance or function (eg, "It's black" or "It holds that thing on your arm," for watchband) are incorrect. Education and socioeconomic factors may influence naming performance, but most individuals should name most of the items effortlessly.

Temporoparietal tasks. A brief sequence of commands can assess language comprehension, ideomotor praxis, and

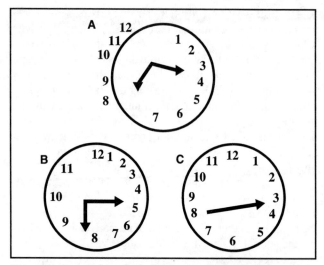

Figure 2: Examples of Clock Drawing Test performance in patients with mild Alzheimer's disease and MMSE score >20. Error types are (A) errors in depicting clock face, numbers, and hands; (B) errors depicting numbers and hands; and (C) errors in representing hands.

left-right orientation. These functions localize to the posterior temporal lobe and inferior parietal lobe, primarily in the left hemisphere. Because AD typically affects these regions of the brain, impaired performance on these tasks strongly supports the diagnosis of AD. If naming is impaired, performance of these tests may not be necessary because anomia generally indicates dysfunction in similar temporal lobe regions.

The patient should be asked to carry out a different imagined action with each hand, eg, using a hammer to hit a nail or a key to open a lock. A subsequent 2-handed task, such as slicing bread, tests the patient's ability to integrate the actions of both hemispheres in a single, spatially specific task. These 3 commands can be followed by tasks that re-

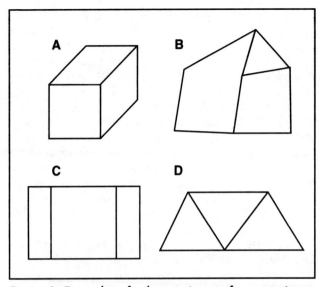

Figure 3: Examples of cube-copying performance in patients with mild and moderate Alzheimer's disease. Copy (A) depicts normal performance, but the patients in copies (B), (C), and (D) fail to capture the 3-dimensional aspects of the image. MMSE scores are (A) 30/30, (B) 26/30, (C) 18/30, and (D) 7/30.

quire the patient to correctly identify right and left, both in reference to his or her own body (eg, "Touch your right hand to your left ear") and the examiner's (eg, "Point to my left hand with your left hand"). Finally, language comprehension for syntactically complex instructions should be tested with a 2-step command in which the word order does not reflect the order of the intended action (eg, "Before pointing to the door, point to the ceiling"). Normal adults will perform all 6 commands flawlessly. Mildly affected AD patients most often perform poorly on the 2-handed praxis test and the syntactically complex command.

Visual constructions. The integration of motor behavior in space is further tested with a drawing task and a copying task. The Clock Drawing Test (CDT) assesses multiple realms of cognition, including executive function (planning), spatial relationships, and semantic knowledge.[9] Many conflicting studies have been published about the utility of the CDT as a screening instrument but, when used in conjunction with other cognitive assessments, it can provide valuable information. Normal performance is placing all numbers and the hands in the correct position. One error is neither sufficiently specific nor sensitive to be useful, but 2 or more errors in placement of the hands carries a predictive value for dementia above 90%.[10] Figure 2 depicts types of abnormalities on clock drawing in mild AD.

Figure copying is another useful visuoconstructive task. Many patients with AD have problems in 3-dimensional processing and depth perception.[11] Asking patients to copy a drawing of a cube or other simple 3-dimensional figure assesses their abilities in cognition. Normal performance is to accurately depict 3 sides and 3 dimensions. Even mildly affected patients with AD may represent 3 visible surfaces with no attempt to show their 3-dimensional relationship (Figure 3).

Memory. After the drawings are completed, the patient should be asked to recall the 3 memory probes. Normal performance is to recall all 3. For those that the patient cannot remember, further steps may clarify the nature of the memory impairment. The patient can be given a semantic clue, such as "One of the words was a kind of flower." Some individuals with poor memory, but not dementia, may need this kind of cueing. They typically respond well to the cues. If the patient's recall is not helped by cueing, the next step is to test recognition memory. For this assessment, the patient is asked to pick the memory probe from a list of semantically related words, eg, "Did I ask you to remember rose, tulip, or daisy?" If a patient requires recognition lists, a memory problem exists severe enough to warrant further testing.

What to Do With the Results of Screening

This screening examination is focused on the expected deficits of AD. If portions of the testing are performed abnormally, then more detailed evaluation for possible AD is required. Because of patients' poor self-monitoring and frequent unawareness of deficits in dementia, permission should be obtained to contact the closest family member for more detailed historical information. Remember that patients with primarily dysexecutive cognitive deficits or behavioral abnormalities may do well on structured tests of cognition, and that further work-up should not be withheld if the history suggests problems in these areas. When the screening is abnormal or further history reveals problems not evident on screening, more evaluation is usually required before a diagnosis of a specific dementing illness can be made.

The further evaluation generally requires a detailed neurologic examination, quantitative measures of cognitive performance, laboratory testing, and imaging. A common complaint of primary care providers is that these portions of the dementia evaluation are too time-consuming. Abnormal cognitive screening is certainly a sufficient indication for referral to a specialist, such as a geriatrician, neurologist or psychiatrist, for diagnosis and treatment recommendations. Hospital-based geriatric assessment or dementia centers that provide this service are available in many communities. Unfortunately, providers and patients may face strong financial disincentives for referrals. Patients also often prefer to maintain their relationships with primary care providers rather than enter a new health-care system.

Consequently, performing the dementia evaluation will often be the responsibility of the primary care provider. Deferring further evaluation and management because of time constraints often backfires. Families expect their primary care provider to recognize health problems and provide guidance

Table 6: The Mini-Mental State Examination (MMSE)*

Orientation

Time: What is the:

1. day of the week ....
2. date ....
3. month ....
4. season ....
5. year ....

Place: Where are we now?

6. address or name of building ....
7. floor ....
8. city ....
9. county ....
10. state ....

Registration

Repeat and remember these 3 words:

11. apple ....
12. table ....
13. penny ....

Repeat as many times as necessary for patient to recall all 3. Score based only on first attempt.

*Used with permission, Folstein MF, Folstein SE, McHugh PR: "Mini-Mental State." A practical method for grading the cognitive state of patients for the clinician. *J Psychiatr Res* 1975;12(3):189-198.

Attention/Calculation

Count backwards from 100 by sevens	or	Spell WORLD backwards
14. 93		14. D ....
15. 86		15. L ....
16. 79		16. R ....
17. 72		17. O ....
18. 65		18. W ....

Recall

Ask patient to recall 3 memory words:

19. apple ....

20. table ....

21. penny ....

Language

Naming: Ask patient to name these items:

22. watch ....

23. pencil ....

Ask patient to follow these instructions: "Take this paper in your right hand, fold it in half, and put it on the floor."

24. uses right hand ....

25. folds in half ....

26. places on floor ....

(continued on next page)

Table 6: The Mini-Mental State Examination (MMSE) *(continued)*

Ask patient to repeat the phrase "No ifs, ands, or buts"

27. repeats correctly ....

Show patient written command "Close your eyes."
Ask patient to do what the paper says.

28. closes eyes ....

Ask patient to write a sentence.

29. writes sentence that contains subject
    and verb and makes sense
    (ignore spelling) ....

Visuospatial

Ask patient to copy the design drawn below.

30. copies correctly (ie, 5 sides for each element);
    polygon at intersections has exactly
    4 sides.

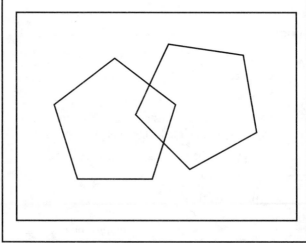

Table 7: Age- and Education-Adjusted Norms for MMSE Performance

These were derived from a random community sample that was not screened for dementia. Based on the epidemiology of AD, the older age groups are likely to include a higher proportion of subjects with dementia. Patients with MMSE scores below the 25th percentile should be considered for more detailed testing to identify possible dementia.

		Age			
Education (yrs)		**60-64**	**70-74**	**80-84**	**>85**
5-8	Median	27	26	25	24
	25th percentile	24	24	22	21
9-12	Median	28	28	26	26
	25th percentile	27	26	23	23
>12	Median	29	29	28	28
	25th percentile	28	27	26	25

Source: Crum et al, 1993.[14]

about what will happen in the future. Much more time and effort will likely be put into crisis management if the patient and family are unclear about the existence of problems and what to expect as dementia progresses. Also, families will leave the patient-provider relationship to find a clinician who better meets their needs. Finally, since effective pharmacologic therapies are available for the treatment of AD, deferring diagnosis may delay the patient's access to optimal care and raise the possibility of litigation.

Table 8: Geriatric Depression Scale (GDS)* (short form)

Patients are asked to respond to the following questions. It may be provided on paper for self-administration. Scores >5 indicate significant depressive symptoms consistent with minor depression and may suggest an indication for therapy.

Choose the best answer for how you felt over the past week:

1. Are you basically satisfied with your life? .... yes/no

2. Have you dropped many of your activities and interests? .... yes/no

3. Do you feel that your life is empty? .... yes/no

4. Do you often get bored? .... yes/no

5. Are you in good spirits most of the time? .... yes/no

6. Are you afraid that something bad is going to happen to you? .... yes/no

7. Do you feel happy most of the time? .... yes/no

*Used with permission, Sheikh JI, Yesavage JA: *Clinical Gerontologist* 1986;5:165-173.

A 'Procedure Visit' Approach to Further Evaluation

When a clinician identifies a problem with a general medical screening test—for instance, a positive stool guaiac test—further testing is almost always indicated. The provider does not generally perform these more detailed tests or procedures at the screening visit. The patient may be referred to a specialist, or the physician may schedule a visit specifically for

8. Do you often feel helpless? .... yes/no

9. Do you prefer to stay at home, rather than going out and doing new things?...... yes/no

10. Do you feel you have more problems with memory than most? .... yes/no

11. Do you think it is wonderful to be alive now? .... yes/no

12. Do you feel pretty worthless the way you are now? .... yes/no

13. Do you feel full of energy? .... yes/no

14. Do you feel that your situation is hopeless? .... yes/no

15. Do you think that most people are better off than you are? .... yes/no

The following answers count 1 point:

1. no	6. yes	11. no
2. yes	7. no	12. yes
3. yes	8. yes	13. no
4. yes	9. yes	14. yes
5. no	10. yes	15. yes

the testing, such as sigmoidoscopy, because of occult stool blood. Therefore, when screening evidence of cognitive or behavioral impairment is identified, the patient can be scheduled for a subsequent extended visit devoted to the procedures necessary for more exact diagnosis and optimal management. Billing and reimbursement regulations vary by health care system and specialty, but procedure codes are available for extended service as well as for psychologic or

Table 9: Functional Activities Questionnaire (FAQ)

A total score for the FAQ is computed by simply summing up the scores across the 10 items. Scores can range from 0 to 30. A cutpoint of '9' (dependent on 3 or more activities) is recommended. If the patient has never

	Never did this
1. Has the patient ever written checks, paid bills, or balanced the checkbook?	X
2. Has the patient ever assembled tax records, business affairs, or papers?	X
3. Has the patient ever shopped alone for clothes, household necessities, or groceries?	X
4. Has the patient ever played a game of skill or worked on a hobby?	X
5. Has the patient ever heated water, made a cup of coffee, or turned off a stove?	X
6. Has the patient ever prepared a balanced meal?	X
7. Has the patient ever kept track of current events?	X
8. Has the patient ever paid attention to, understood, or discussed TV, books, or magazines?	X
9. Does the patient remember appointments, family occasions, holidays, or when to take medications?	X
10. Has the patient ever traveled out of neighborhood, driven, or arranged to take buses?	X

done the task, ask the informant to estimate the level of the patient's performance and mark the *Never did this* item to document that this is an estimate.

Is (would be) dependent on others	Can (could) do with assistance	Has (would have) difficulty but does by self	Is (would be) normal
3	2	1	0
3	2	1	0
3	2	1	0
3	2	1	0
3	2	1	0
3	2	1	0
3	2	1	0
3	2	1	0
3	2	1	0
3	2	1	0

Pfeffer RT et al: *J Gerontol* 1982;37:323-329. Copyright© The Gerontological Society of America. Reproduced by permission of the publisher.

Table 10: Physical Self-Maintenance Scale (PSMS) for Activities of Daily Living

Numbers 1 through 5 in each category represent worsening states of function. The clinician should choose the number that best describes the patient's functional status. Scores in all 6 categories are totaled. The higher the final score, the greater the degree of impairment.

A. Toileting

1. Cares for self at toilet completely, no incontinence.
2. Needs to be reminded or needs help in cleaning self, or has rare (weekly at most) accidents.
3. Soiling or wetting while asleep more than once a week.
4. Soiling or wetting while awake more than once a week.
5. No control of bowels or bladder.

B. Feeding

1. Eats without assistance.
2. Eats with minor assistance at mealtimes and/or with special preparation of food, or help in cleaning up after meals.
3. Feeds self with moderate assistance and is untidy.
4. Requires extensive assistance for all meals.
5. Does not feed self at all and resists efforts of others to feed him/her.

C. Dressing

1. Dresses, undresses, and selects clothes from own wardrobe.
2. Dresses and undresses self with minor assistance.
3. Needs moderate assistance in dressing or selection of clothes.
4. Needs major assistance in dressing, but cooperates with efforts of others to help.
5. Completely unable to dress self and resists efforts of others to help.

D. Grooming (neatness, hair, nails, hands, face, clothing)

1. Always neatly dressed, well groomed, without assistance.
2. Grooms self adequately with occasional minor assistance, eg, shaving.
3. Needs moderate and regular assistance or supervision in grooming.
4. Needs total grooming care, but can remain well groomed after help from others.
5. Actively negates all efforts of others to maintain grooming.

Lawton MP, Brody EM: *Gerontologist* 1969;9:179-186.

(continued on next page)

Table 10: Physical Self-Maintenance Scale (PSMS) for Activities of Daily Living
(continued)

E. Physical Ambulation

1. Goes about grounds or city.

2. Ambulates within residence or about one-block distance.

3. Ambulates with assistance of (check one)

   a ( ) another person

   b ( ) railing

   c ( ) cane

   d ( ) walker

   e ( ) wheelchair—gets in and out without help

   f ( ) wheelchair—needs help getting in and/or out.

4. Sits unsupported in chair or wheelchair, but cannot propel self without help.

5. Bedridden more than half the time.

F. Bathing

1. Bathes self (tub, shower, sponge bath) without help.

2. Bathes self with help getting in and out of tub.

3. Washes face and hands only, but cannot bathe rest of body.

4. Does not wash self, but is cooperative with those who bathe him/her.

5. Does not try to wash self, and resists efforts to keep him/her clean.

TOTAL

neuropsychologic testing by the physician. Cost-effective diagnosis of dementing illnesses is facilitated by the proper use of these CPT codes.[12]

Standardized Instruments

The use of procedure codes for psychologic testing generally requires the administration of 2 or more standardized instruments. For dementia assessment, these should uniformly include a quantitative measure of cognition. The Mini-Mental State Examination,[13] illustrated in Table 6, is the most commonly used. It has the advantage of being familiar to many providers, which allows a quick shorthand means of communicating severity information to consultants and other care providers. It is broken down into domains to help interpret areas of strength and weakness in cognition. In addition, there are published norms that facilitate adjustment for the influences of age and education on performance (Table 7).[14]

The MMSE is not perfect for the diagnosis of dementia, particularly the non-Alzheimer's forms. Fully one third of the score is based on orientation to time and place, while there are only cursory assessments of language and praxis. In addition, the 5 (out of the 30) points assessing attention and concentration can be assessed in quite different ways. Most patients with dementia, and many healthy older adults, find the serial subtraction of sevens to be much more difficult than spelling 'world' in reverse order. This ambiguity can lead to wide variations in administration of the questions and interpretation of the results. Despite these weaknesses, it remains the most broadly accepted and best characterized brief measure of cognitive abilities.

Some clinicians may prefer to use the Blessed Orientation-Memory-Concentration test[15] or the Short Portable Mental Status Questionnaire.[16] Other useful information about mood state and function can be derived from the modified Geriatric Depression Scale (GDS)[17] (Table 8), the Functional Activities Questionnaire (FAQ)[18] (Table 9), and the Physical Self Maintenance Scale (PSMS)[19] (Table 10). These and other standardized assessment scales for use in dementia have been compiled by Herndon[20] and in the AHCPR Quick Reference Guide.[2] The primary value of standardized scales is to develop quantitative or objective measures of cognition, behavior, and function that can be used to assess progression of illness and response to treatment.

Additional Mental State Characterization

Screening and quantitative evaluations usually provide enough information to make a diagnosis of AD. Differentiating other dementia types may require more extensive cognitive evaluation. This section will briefly review other testing that may be useful at the bedside. More detail on how to perform and interpret tests of cognitive function is available in Strub and Black.[21] Current billing practices and regulations generally allow for reimbursement of a detailed mental state examination when documentation clearly shows the procedures are in excess of standard assessments.

Orientation. If orientation to time and place is not assessed as part of a quantified instrument, it should be checked. Many patients with dementia try to minimize aspects of disorientation with excuses like, "I didn't look at the paper today" or "I'm retired so the days don't matter much to me." These statements are red flags for significant disorientation. Further questioning might include inquiries about the approximate time of day, what meal might be expected next, or what the last major holiday was. Disorientation to self occurs only in advanced dementia. Its presence in the context of mild or moderate cognitive disability suggests delirium or a primary psychiatric disturbance.

Memory. Learning and short-term memory are assessed in the cognitive screening, but other aspects of memory can also be tested. Remote memory can be checked by asking the patient to list, in reverse order, the last 5 presidents. If the information can be confirmed by a knowledgeable informant, patients might be asked when they were married (or widowed), how many grandchildren they have (and their ages), or to recount their military service or employment history.

Spatial memory can be assessed in the office by asking the patient to observe while the clinician identifies and hides an object in the examination room, such as showing a watch or stethoscope to the patient and then placing it in a drawer. The physical or cognitive examination continues for a few minutes and then the patient is asked to recall what was hidden (object memory) and where (spatial memory).

Since details are lost from remote memory in AD, it may be useful to ask the patient to recall his or her own experiences of important historical events, such as the Pearl Harbor attack, the JFK assassination, and the September 11, 2001, terrorist attacks in the U.S. It is impossible to know how accurately the patient recalls the experience, but adults with intact memories are usually able to give lucid and richly detailed recollections of how they received the news, how they reacted, who they were with, etc. Those with poor memories will often be very vague or give temporally inappropriate replies, eg, hearing of Pearl Harbor at work or on television.

Frontal/executive function. This aspect of cognition can be difficult to test. Controlled oral word association can provide useful information. In this test, the patient is asked to state as many words as he or she can that conform to a category set by the examiner. This is a common neuropsychologic test that can be abbreviated for use in a medical assessment. The first category is words that start with a particular letter, often 'f' or 's.' Before starting, patients should be told that neither proper nouns nor variations of the same root word (fly, flew, flying, etc) will be counted. The number of words produced in 1 minute is recorded. The second part of the test follows immediately. In this section, the patient is asked to produce as many words as possible that fit a semantic category, such as animals or fruits. Cognitively intact individuals generally find the semantic task to be easier and produce a longer

Table 11: Key Elements of the Neurologic Examination in the Clinical Approach to Dementia (Excluding Mental State)

Cranial Nerves:

  II. Optic nerve: visual fields, retinal changes

  III, IV, VI. Ocular motor nerves: pupillary reflex, extraocular movements

  V. Trigeminal: facial sensation

  VII. Facial: facial movement and symmetry

  VIII. Vestibular: hearing symmetry

  IX. Glossopharyngeal: palate elevation and symmetry

  XI. Spinal accessory: shoulder shrug symmetry and power

  XII. Hypoglossal: tongue protrusion

Motor Function:

- Power
- Tone
  - limbs
  - neck
- Abnormal movements
  - myoclonus
  - tremor

list on that task. Producing more words on the letter-based list suggests a problem with semantics and supports a diagnosis of AD. In contrast, the person with more prominent executive function deficits often produces short word lists on both parts of the task. The single-letter form of the test is not well standardized, but an intact adult with a

Tendon Reflexes:

- Symmetry
- Proximal vs distal
- Lateralized hyperreflexia

Pathologic Reflexes:

- Plantar (Babinski)
- Grasp

Sensation:

- Symmetry
- Distal sensation
  - proprioception
  - vibration
  - pain/temperature

Coordination:

- Rapid movements
- Ataxia

Gait:

- Postural stability
- Stride length
- Gait initiation

high school education can be expected to generate a list of at least 10 to 12 words.

The antisaccade test assesses the patient's ability to resist distraction. In this test, the examiner instructs the patient to establish ocular fixation on the examiner's nose and then make volitional eye movements to targets in peripheral vi-

Table 12: American Academy of Neurology Guidelines for Blood Testing in the Assessment of Dementia[3]

Recommended:

- Complete blood count
- Serum electrolytes (including calcium)
- Glucose
- BUN/Creatinine
- Liver function tests
- Thyroid function tests
- Vitamin B_{12} level

Optional:

- Syphilis serology
- Erythrocyte sedimentation rate
- Serum folate
- HIV (per Centers for Disease Control protocol)

sion, typically the examiner's wiggling fingers. Subsequently, the patient is informed that the 'rules are going to change.' The patient is once again asked to fixate on the examiner's nose, but is instructed to look to the hand that stays still when the other one is moving. The movements are repeated over a series of trials, usually 5 times per side. Intact performance requires that the patient withhold a reflexive response to a moving peripheral visual target and execute a motor program in the opposite direction. Patients with impaired executive regulation of behavior will often fail to suppress the reflexive saccadic eye movement or demonstrate a prolonged delay before refixating in the proper direction.

Another test of frontal function was developed by the Russian psychologist Luria. In this test, the examiner demonstrates a 3-step motor sequence with one hand. The examiner taps a fist, then the palm of the same hand, and then the hypothenar edge of the hand on his or her own leg and continues to repeat the same 3 postures. The patient is asked to mimic the pattern as the examiner continues. After several repeats with the patient, the examiner stops and observes how well the patient is able to sustain the pattern. It is important that verbal labels for the postures not be used, because this facilitates performance of the task. If the task is performed correctly, the patient can be asked to transfer the motor pattern to the other hand. Not all healthy older adults can perform this task, but those with frontal or executive impairments often struggle significantly. Strub and Black[21] provide more detailed accounts of performing and interpreting bedside tests in this complex cognitive realm.

Abstraction. Abstract reasoning is impaired in many forms of dementia. This can be assessed by asking the patient to identify abstract similarities in word pairs, eg, "How is a chair like a table?" or "How is an apple like a banana?" People with dementia are apt to note the difference rather than a similarity. Alternatively, they are likely to identify a concrete rather than abstract similarity. Examples of concrete responses would include that a chair and table 'go together' or that the apple and banana 'have skin.' Interpretation of proverbs is another task of abstract reasoning that can be used at the bedside but is less desirable because of cultural and educational biases.

Attention and concentration. To test these related parts of cognition, the patient can be asked to perform reversals, such as stating the days of the week or the months in reverse order. Digit span is a test of primary memory that also depends on attention. In this task, the patient is asked to repeat a string of random digits in the order that he or she heard them. Normal performance is to repeat strings of 5 or more correctly. Deficits may be more pronounced when patients are asked to repeat digits in reverse order.

Table 13: Red Flags for Potential AD on MDS Full Assessment

Section B. Cognitive Patterns

2. Memory	Memory problems identified on either short or long term
3. Memory/Recall	Any checked box
4. Cognitive Skills	Any score > 0
5. Indicators of Delirium	Score of 1 on any section

Section C. Communication/Hearing

4. Making Self Understood	Any score > 0
6. Ability to Understand	Scores of 2 or 3 (as long as hearing score = 0-1)

Section D. Mood and Behavior Patterns

1. Indications of Depression/Anxiety/Sad Mood

  b. repetitive questions

  f. unrealistic fears

  i. repetitive non-health concerns   Any score > 0 on these items

  n. repetitive physical movements

  o. withdrawal from activities/interests

  p. reduced social interaction

4. Behavioral Symptoms	Any score > 0

Section F. Psychosocial Well-Being

1. Sense of Initiative — Checks *absent* for items c or d

2. Unsettled Relationships — Checks *present* for items e or g

Section G. Physical Functioning and Structural Problems

1. ADL Self Performance

    g. dressing
    i. toilet use
    j. personal hygiene — Any score > 0 for self performance (when not clearly related to physical disability)

7. Task Segmentation — Score of 1

Section K. Oral/Nutritional Status

3. Weight Change — Score of 1 for weight loss

Section N. Activity/Pursuit Patterns

2. Time in Activities — Scores of 2 or 3

5. Change in Activities — Score of 0

Section O. Medications

Days Received Medication

    a. antipsychotic — Any score > 0

    b. antianxiety — Any progressive increase in score

Table 14: Cognitive Performance Scale Scores Range From 0 (No Dementia) to 6 (Very Severe Dementia)

MDS Section:

B-1   Comatose

        0 - No   1 - Yes

B-2a   Short-Term Memory - OK, seems/appears to recall after 5 minutes

        0 - Memory OK   1 - Memory problem

B-4   Cognition Skills for Daily Decision Making (Made decisions regarding tasks of daily life in previous 7 days)

        0 - Independent - decisions are consistent/reasonable

        1 - Modified independence - some difficulty in new situations only

        2 - Moderately impaired - decisions poor; cues/supervision required

        3 - Severely impaired - never/rarely made decisions

Normal performance in this task is to reach a span at least 2 digits less than the forward span.

Language. In addition to the naming and command-following assessed in the screening examination, other parts of language function should be evaluated. These include the fluency and effortfulness of speech, sentence

C-4   Communication/Hearing Patterns - Making Self Understood (Expressing information content, however able)

0 - Understood

1 - Usually understood - difficulty finding words or finishing thoughts

2 - Sometimes understood - ability is limited to making concrete requests

3 - Rarley/never understood

G-1h   Physical Functioning and Structural Problems

Eating: How resident eats and drinks (regardless of skill). Includes intake of nourishment by other means (eg, tube feeding, TPN)

0 - No help/Set up from staff

1 – Set-up help only

2 - One person physical assist

3 - Two + persons physical assist

8 - ADL activity itself did not occur during entire 7 days

repetition, reading, and writing. All are accomplished competently in the healthy older adult. Impairments in fluency or repetition raise the possibility of frontotemporal dementia or a vascular lesion in the language-dominant hemisphere. Impairments in reading (with intact visual acuity) suggest visual association cortex dysfunction, as is seen in posterior cortical atrophy or the visual variant of Alzheimer's disease.

Neurologic Examination

A thorough neurologic examination is always indicated as a part of the evaluation of dementia. Particular emphasis should be placed on assessment for focal findings in the central nervous system, such as visual field deficits, hemiparesis, hemisensory loss, reflex asymmetries, and Babinski's sign. Extrapyramidal dysfunction, such as rigidity or bradykinesia, and gait disorders are more difficult to discern from healthy aging but provide important information in the differential diagnosis of dementia. Clinicians should pay particular attention to the patient's ability to initiate gait and take normal strides. Postural reflexes can be assessed with the examiner standing behind the patient and briskly, but gently, pulling back on the patient's shoulders. Healthy adults may take 1 or 2 small steps to right themselves. Impaired righting reflexes, such as those seen in many extrapyramidal syndromes, will manifest as falling or retropulsion toward the examiner. Key elements of the neurologic examination are depicted in Table 11.

Laboratory Testing

The American Academy of Neurology has published practice guidelines that include recommendations for the laboratory evaluation of dementia. These include assessing the general health of the patient with a comprehensive blood chemistry panel (eg, Chem-20) and a complete blood count. These tests are most useful for determining systemic illnesses that might be causing or exacerbating cognitive impairment. Testing is also recommended for specific treatable disease states that cause dementia, including hypothyroidism, and vitamin B_{12} deficiency. Past recommendations requiring routine screening for neurosyphilis have been superseded. Now, syphilis screening can be considered similar to other tests such as lumbar puncture, heavy metal screening, or HIV testing, depending on the patient's clinical profile and the recognition of appropriate risk factors. The AAN laboratory evaluation guidelines are shown in Table 12. AD-specific laboratory assessments, as well as imaging and other adjuncts to diagnosis, are addressed in Chapter 6.

Detecting AD in Residential Care

The previous sections of this chapter focus on the assessment of patients living in the community alone or with family members. Patients residing in residential care facilities may require a different approach to diagnosis, depending on the severity of dementia and the information available. Only a minority of dementia patients live in residential care settings, such as assisted-living facilities, rest homes, group homes, and nursing homes. However, a higher proportion of the residential population will have dementia, and this will include more of those classified as severely demented. In these environments, the staff, rather than family caregivers, may be called upon to recognize patterns of cognitive or behavioral change that signal dementia. In the past, late detection had little impact because no specific pharmacotherapy was available for AD. However, with growing evidence that drug treatments may provide benefit into the later stages of dementia, there is likely to be an increased emphasis on diagnosis and treatment of AD in residential care.

Using the MDS to Trigger
Medical Evaluation for Dementia

Many of the techniques described above for use in ambulatory settings apply to more mildly affected people in residential care. The scope of assessment and uniform use of the federally mandated Minimum Data Set (MDS) in institutional long-term care make this instrument a useful adjunct for detecting dementia in these settings. To be reliable as a dementia screening tool, MDS evaluators must consider the patient's function in the context of appropriate expectations for age, education, and socioeconomic status for the population as a whole, and not just the residents under their care. This helps to avoid underdetection of dementia due to the 'normality' of dementia-related behaviors in residential settings. If a high proportion of the professionals' case load has dementia their perception of what is typical for age may become skewed.

Several sections of the MDS can provide crucial information for detecting incipient dementia not recorded in the diagnosis list (Table 13). Sections on cognition (B), communication/hearing (C), mood and behavior (E), psychosocial well-being (F), physical functioning (G), oral/nutrition status (K), activities/pursuits (N), and medications (O) can provide information that suggests dementia even when it is not coded in the disease diagnoses section (I). Table 13 lists key sections that suggest possible dementia from the MDS full assessment form. Many of these sections call for assessment of changes over the last 90 days. Unfortunately, 3 months may be too short a period to detect progression of early AD. Questions of similar content are also a part of the MDS quarterly assessment form.

A standardized cognitive performance scale has also been developed from the MDS and is known as the MDS-CPS (Table 14). This scale correlates closely with the MiniMental State examination in identifying dementia, with an overall diagnostic accuracy of 96%.[22,23] MDS-CPS scores suggesting dementia should trigger the treating physician to evaluate for possible AD.

Pharmacy Records

Another potential source for identifying incipient dementia is medication usage. Many residential clients have standing PRN orders that range from laxatives to anxiolytics and hypnotics. A change in usage patterns for PRN psychotropic agents may suggest that family members or nursing staff have identified emerging behavioral changes that warrant intervention. Because the order is pre-existing, the staff may not closely document the patient's change in behavior or report it to the physician until the severity exceeds the ability of the standing order to manage it.

References

1. McKhann G, Drachman D, Folstein M, et al: Clinical diagnosis of Alzheimer's disease: report of the NINCDS-ADRDA work group under the auspices of the Department of Health and Human Services Task Force on Alzheimer's disease. *Neurology* 1984;34:939-944.

2. Costa PT Jr, Williams TF, Somerfeld M, et al: Early identification of Alzheimer's Disease and related dementias. *Clinical Practice Guideline, Quick Reference Guide for Clinicians*, No. 19. Rockville, MD, US Department of Health and Human Services, Public Health Service, Agency for Health Care Policy and Research, AHCPR Publication No. 97-0703, November 1996.

3. Knopman DS, DeKosky ST, Cummings JL, et al: Practice parameter: diagnosis of dementia (an evidence-based review). Report of the Quality Standards Subcommittee of the American Academy of Neurology. *Neurology* 2001;56:1143-1153.

4. Corey-Bloom J, Thal L, Galasko D, et al: Diagnosis and evaluation of dementia. *Neurology* 1995;45:211-218.

5. American Psychiatric Association practice guideline for the treatment of patients with Alzheimer's disease and other dementias of late life. *Am J Psychiatry* 1997;154:1-39.

6. Small GW, Rabins PV, Barry PB, et al: Diagnosis and treatment of Alzheimer's disease and related disorders: consensus statement of the American Association for Geriatric Psychiatry, the Alzheimer's Association, and the American Geriatrics Society. *JAMA* 1997;278:1363-1371.

7. Clarfield AM: The reversible dementias: do they reverse? *Ann Intern Med* 1988;109:476-486.

8. Jacobs DM, Sano M, Dooneif G, et al: Neuropsychological detection and characterization of preclinical Alzheimer's disease. *Neurology* 1995;45:957-962.

9. Mendez MF, Ala T, Underwood KL: Development of scoring criteria for the clock drawing task in Alzheimer's disease. *J Am Geriatr Soc* 1992;40:1095-1099.

10. Esteban-Santillan C, Praditsuwan R, Ueda H, et al: Clock drawing test in very mild Alzheimer's disease. *J Am Geriatr Soc* 1998; 46:1266-1269.

11. Mendez MF, Mendez MA, Martin R, et al: Complex visual disturbances in Alzheimer's disease. *Neurology* 1990;40:439-443.

12. Geldmacher DS: Cost effective recognition and diagnosis of dementia. *Semin Neurology* 2002;22:63-70.

13. Folstein MF, Folstein SE, McHugh PR, et al: "Mini-mental state." A practical method of grading cognitive state of patients for the clinician. *J Psychiatr Res* 1975;12:189-198.

14. Crum RM, Anthony JC, Bassett SS, et al: Population-based norms for the Mini-Mental State Examination by age and education level. *JAMA* 1993;269:2386-2391.

15. Katzman R, Brown T, Fuld P, et al: Validation of a short Orientation-Memory-Concentration Test of cognitive impairment. *Am J Psychiatry* 1983;140:734-739.

16. Pfeiffer E: A short portable mental status questionnaire for the assessment of organic brain deficit in elderly patients. *J Am Geriatr Soc* 1975;23:433-441.

17. Sheikh JI, Yesavage JA: Geriatric Depression Scale (GDS): Recent evidence and development of a shorter version. *Clin Gerontol* 1986;5:165-173.

18. Pfeffer RI, Kurosaki TT, Harrah CH, et al: Measurement of functional activities in older adults in the community. *J Gerontol* 1982;37:323-329.

19. Lawton MP, Brody EM: Assessment of older people: self-maintaining and instrumental activities of daily living. *Gerontologist* 1969;9:179-186.

20. Herndon RM, ed: *Handbook of Neurologic Rating Scales*. New York, Demos Vermande, 1997.

21. Strub RL, Black FW: *The Mental Status Examination in Neurology*, 3rd ed. Philadelphia, FA Davis, 1993.

22. Hartmaier SL, Sloane PD, Guess HA, et al: Validation of the Minimum Data Set Cognitive Performance Scale: agreement with the MiniMental State Examination. *J Gerontology* (Series A). Biological Sciences and Medical Science. 1995;50:M128-M133.

23. Morris JN, Fries BE, Mehr DR, et al: MDS Cognitive Performance Scale. *J Gerontology* 1994:49:M174-182.

Chapter 6

Supporting Clinical Diagnosis

I n some cases, the clinical approach to dementia diagnosis outlined in Chapter 5 will not be sufficient to provide a satisfactory explanation for the cause of cognitive complaints. This chapter reviews how other testing can improve diagnostic certainty. These procedures need not be considered a routine part of all evaluations, nor should they be used as alternatives to carefully considered clinical diagnosis.

Anatomic Imaging

Significant controversy exists over whether all patients presenting with dementia should receive a diagnostic imaging test of the brain. The American Academy of Neurology (AAN) practice guidelines now consider imaging to be a recommended procedure.[1] In routine practice, brain imaging is used to determine whether any structural lesions of the brain are causing, or more likely contributing to, the cognitive disturbance. The primary goal of anatomic imaging is to identify reversible sources of dementia, like those depicted in Table 1. For any person presenting with neurologic examination findings that localize to a specific brain region, the efficacy of imaging has been supported.[2] In addition, because the likelihood of successful reversal of impairment is highest in patients with early, mild, atypical, or rapidly changing neurobehavioral profiles, these patients also warrant imaging in most cases.

The choice of x-ray computed tomography (CT) vs magnetic resonance imaging (MRI) should be dictated by the clinical circumstances. For example, CT without contrast enhancement will reliably detect hydrocephalus, but not necessarily predict treatment response (Chapter 4). Although contrast enhancement with iodine-based injections will improve CT's ability to detect subdural hematoma and meningioma, the likelihood of significant cognitive compromise in the absence of brain deformation detectable on uncontrasted CT is quite low. MRI offers better spatial resolution than CT, but is more uncomfortable to the patient (especially patients with claustrophobia), costs more, and the results take longer to obtain. Because many dementia patients have difficulty remembering and cooperating with instructions to lie still, MRI's longer acquisition time makes it more prone to movement artifacts. This leads to repeat procedures and increased cost as well as to delays in diagnosis. Therefore, for most routine dementia evaluations, uncontrasted CT is appropriate.

Apart from cerebral atrophy, which is nonspecific, the most common finding on imaging is white matter rarefaction, also called leukoaraiosis.[3] This is often interpreted as evidence for cerebrovascular disease, but the clinician must be cautious in assuming that the white

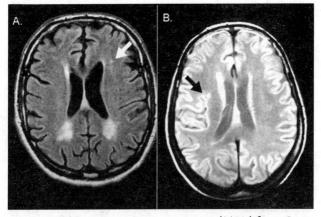

Figure 1: Magnetic resonance images (MRIs) from 2 patients. Image A is from an 83-year-old man with typical age-related memory complaints but normal daily function, and Mini-Mental State Examination (MMSE) scores of 28/30 and 29/30, 1 year apart. Image B is from a 72-year-old woman with dementia of undetermined etiology that prevents her from living independently. Her MMSE declined from 24 to 19 in 1 year of follow-up. These images reflect the nonspecific nature of periventricular white matter change and focal hyperintensities (see arrows) on MRI in the older adult population.

matter findings are causing dementia. Overinterpretation of white matter changes, especially on MRI, leads to overdiagnosis of vascular dementia (VaD). Changes in white matter are most clearly associated with aging and with chronic hypertension, but their relationship with cognitive impairment is low.[4,5] In fact, 30% to 90% of cognitively intact older adults will have nonspecific white matter disease evident on T2-weighted MRI.[6] Figure 1 demonstrates typical MRI in older adults with and without dementia. If the intent of imaging is to identify strokes that support a diagnosis of VaD, focal lucencies on CT or T1-weighted MRI are far more specific and, therefore, more clinically useful.

Regardless of the specificity of the radiographic findings for dementia, ischemic cerebrovascular lesions are not reversible. Given the high rates of vasculopathic risk factors in populations expressing dementia, risk-factor management for stroke should be considered in all persons with dementing illnesses, whether imaging reveals possible ischemic change or not.

Neuropsychologic Assessment

Neuropsychologic assessment is closely related to bedside mental state testing, but can provide much richer detail and more structured comparisons to normal and age-matched performance. Neuropsychologists are generally PhD-level licensed psychologists with specific training in cognitive testing procedures and interpretation. Neuropsychologic assessment is based on observation and measurement of an individual's behavior in relation to stimuli selected to provoke an abnormal response in patients with damage in a specific neuroanatomical structure.[7] Physician-based 'bedside' cognitive assessment in the form of mental status testing is generally designed to identify abnormalities associated with disease. This is known as a *pathognomonic* approach. In contrast, many neuropsychologic assessments are designed to evaluate an individual's performance in comparison to an appropriate reference population. This is considered a *normative* approach. A combination of pathognomonic and normative tests is especially useful in characterizing the pattern, severity, and clinical relevance of deficits associated with dementia.

Referral Questions

Neuropsychologic referral in persons with suspected dementia can assist in answering several important questions. Differentiating benign, age-related cognitive compromise from incipient dementia can be an important role for the neuropsychologist. There is, however, considerable overlap in the performance of mildly demented and healthy older adults.[8] A well-conducted neuropsychologic assessment should, therefore, always include a careful history, including information from knowledgeable informants, to place any performance deficiencies observed on testing in the appropriate context.

Differentiating depression from dementia is another question well suited to neuropsychologic testing. This differentiation can be very challenging, however, because depression is a common feature in dementia, as well as an independent cause of cognitive impairment. Generally, most depressed patients will not show generalized cognitive deficits.[9] Deficits in tasks demanding more mental effort are particularly vulnerable to depression. These include the essential elements of bedside testing: learning, free recall, and abstract thinking. Therefore, the more extensive comparison of effortful and noneffortful mental tasks that can be obtained in neuropsychologic assessment can clarify the role of depression in cognitive impairment.

Another role of neuropsychologic assessment is the evaluation of strengths and weaknesses in the cognitive profile to guide management. For instance, identifying a prominent dysexecutive state might lead a clinician to recommend discontinuation of driving or a transition to a more supported living environment. Alternatively, a relative preservation of language comprehension in comparison to expressive speech might be discerned, as occurs in Pick's disease. This would allow the psychologist to counsel the family about appropriate expectations for communicating with the affected patient, or trigger a referral to a speech/language pathologist to develop a communication system that acknowledges the degree of comprehension and compensates for poor expression. Although rarely practical in clinical settings, neuropsychologic testing can be used to measure responses to medications, particularly in domains that fall outside of the cognitive realms feasibly assessed by the prescribing clinician.

Similarly, neuropsychologic assessment can assist in differential diagnosis among dementias. This also involves examining the profile of test results in comparison to reference populations, ideally dementia groups with subsequent postmortem confirmation of clinical diagnosis. For example, one study has suggested that as a group, dementia with Lewy bodies (DLB) patients have more difficulty with visuoperceptual, visuoconstructive, and visuospatial functions, but less of a verbal memory deficit than Alzheimer's disease (AD) patients on neuropsychologic examination.[10] A major shortcoming of this kind of analysis is the fact that any individual patient may vary widely from the average findings for a particular diagnosis. These observations would therefore be inappropriate for differentiating a patient with prominent visual disturbance in AD from a DLB patient with worse-than-average memory loss. Similar difficulties exist for differentiating patients with extensive frontal lobe symptoms in AD from those with frontotemporal dementia. For this reason, no single neuropsychologic test is capable of definitively distinguishing between disease states. Nonetheless, a carefully conducted neuropsychologic evaluation can provide much useful and practical information.

Functional Imaging

Unlike standard anatomic imaging procedures, such as CT or MRI, functional imaging techniques can provide information about the metabolic activity of brain regions. Thus, instead of providing a picture of how the components of the brain *look*, functional imaging attempts to answer questions about how well different brain regions *work*. For clinical purposes, the primary functional imaging methods are the nuclear medicine procedures of positron emission tomography (PET) and single-photon emission computed tomography (SPECT). More recently, magnetic susceptibility functional MRI (fMRI) methods of assessing local cerebral blood volume have been introduced. Along with magnetic resonance spectroscopy, fMRI is primarily a research tool.

SPECT is perhaps the most accessible of these procedures because of easy commercial availability of the radiopharmaceutical Tc-99-HMPAO (technetium-99m hexamethylpropyleneamine oxime). Tc-99-HMPAO crosses the blood-brain barrier and undergoes radioactive decay slowly enough to allow tomographic imaging. The radiographic signals provide information on local blood flow. Because blood flow to the cerebral cortex reflects metabolic demand, cell death and synaptic loss in dementia result in reduced blood flow. SPECT images in Alzheimer's disease generally demonstrate reductions in cortical perfusion in temporal and parietal lobes. High sensitivity (96%) and specificity (89%) for autopsy-verified Alzheimer's disease have been reported.[11] A problem with SPECT scanning is that it correlates closely with symptoms identified on clinical examination, so that the detection of parietal lobe hypoperfusion may be difficult in patients with little aphasia, apraxia, or visuospatial disturbance. Therefore, its diagnostic utility in early or mild patients—in whom supplemental diagnostic testing is most needed—remains questionable.[12] Other patterns detectable on SPECT include frontotemporal hypoperfusion in association with frontal type dementia and patchy areas of hypoperfusion associated with cerebral ischemia in the multi-infarct type of VaD.[13] Depression can also cause frontal hypoperfusion, which may cloud differential diagnosis when it is unclear whether depression is the cause or a complication of cognitive difficulties. In general, a negative SPECT scan argues against AD but does not exclude it. A negative scan therefore raises the likelihood of non-AD dementia.

PET may be used in some institutions capable of making the 'hotter' radioisotopes necessary for this procedure. PET offers the advantage of higher spatial resolution than SPECT and the opportunity to directly measure cellular glucose metabolism with agents like [18]fluorodeoxyglucose (FDG), instead of surrogates like blood flow. PET images have been useful in research questions, such as localizing anatomic regions of dysfunction contributing to visual disturbances in AD,[14] but superiority to SPECT or conventional diagnostic imaging in clinical diagnosis has not been established.

Electroencephalography

The value of electroencephalography (EEG) in the diagnosis of dementia is somewhat controversial. Current practice guidelines consider EEG an optional procedure. In many cases of early AD, routine clinical EEG is unrevealing, because the degree of EEG abnormality generally correlates well with dementia severity. Numerous reports examine group differences between dementia and nondementia groups. However, the key issue of positive and negative predictive values of clinical EEG interpretation for the diagnosis of dementia in *mildly affected* individuals is rarely addressed. For example, moderate to severely abnormal EEGs were found in only half of a group of AD patients with disease duration less than 4 years.[15] This is a very low yield when the 8- to 10-year average survival rate of AD cases is considered. Furthermore, EEG cannot reliably discriminate between the most common causes of dementia.[16] The additive value of EEG is highest when the degree of diagnostic certainty is lowest.[17] Therefore, EEG is unlikely to be of great utility when the clinical pattern matches diagnostic criteria for one of the dementing illnesses. Reasonably specific EEG findings are associated in Creutzfeldt-Jakob disease, acute stroke, hepatic encephalopathy, and nonconvulsive status epilepticus.

Table 2: Genetic Testing in AD

AD Type	Chromosome	Gene
Early-onset familial	21	Amyloid precursor protein (APP)
Early-onset familial	14	Presenilin-1 (PS-1)
Familial (variable onset)	1	Presenilin-2 (PS-2)
Late-onset famial (possibly sporadic)	19	Apolipoprotein ε4 allele (risk factor only)

AD-specific Blood Tests

The ε4 allele of apolipoprotein E (ApoE) is associated with increased risk for AD, especially the late-onset familial forms. Its value in routine clinical diagnosis of dementia is controversial. In one large, multicenter study, the primary utility of finding a patient with an ApoE ε4 allele was a small reduction in false-positive diagnosis of AD.[18] Caution in interpreting this well-performed study is warranted, however, because when most of the clinical and pathologic samples were collected, there was less understanding of dementia with Lewy bodies (DLB). Many cases were therefore interpreted as parkinsonian variants of AD. The finding that ApoE ε4 is also associated with neuropathologically confirmed DLB also clouds the reported diagnostic specificity of ApoE testing.[19] Testing a patient for ApoE status also carries implications for risk among unaffected family members. ApoE testing should therefore be linked to genetic counseling for unaffected (and untested) family members. Several consensus groups have agreed that

ApoE should never be used as a clinical predictive test in asymptomatic individuals.

Early-onset AD cases (ie, onset before ages 50 to 55) frequently present in the context of an autosomal-dominant pattern of inheritance. When family history is unclear, testing for mutations on chromosomes 1 (PS-2), 14 (PS-1), and 21(APP) may be indicated. Because of the implications for family members, especially children of the affected person, this testing should be accomplished only in conjunction with formal genetic counseling. Recognized mutations in any of these genes are present in only a very small minority of all AD cases (< 5%) and less than half of all early-onset, autosomal-dominant, familial cases. Table 2 depicts the known genetic factors in AD for which blood tests are available.

Lumbar Puncture

Lumbar puncture was once a routine part of the evaluation of dementia, but is now considered optional. Generally, for the degree of real or imagined patient discomfort and the practitioner time involved in obtaining cerebrospinal fluid (CSF), the utility of routine CSF examination is low. Most dementia forms are not associated with changes in CSF cell counts, protein, or glucose. If treponemal-specific syphilis blood tests (eg FTA-ABS, MHATP) are positive, CSF examination is warranted to evaluate for the possibility of neurosyphilis. Neurosyphilis that is sufficiently active to be the cause of dementia will be characterized by a positive VDRL or RPR test and by the presence of leukocytosis (at least 5 white blood cells per mm^3) in the CSF. The sensitivity of FTA-ABS and MHATP reduces their value in CSF assessment, because even small amounts of blood contamination of the CSF can result in a false-positive CSF result.

CSF tests for pathophysiologic correlates of AD have been developed. These include assays for the soluble forms of β-amyloid. With increased deposition of insoluble species of amyloid in AD, CSF concentration of β-amyloid, particularly the 42-43 amino acid forms, is reduced.[20] Similarly, the neuronal damage in AD is associated with release of tau protein into the extracellular compartment, leading to increased concentration of tau in the CSF.[21] For neither of these assays alone are the positive and negative predictive values adequate to augment criterion-based clinical diagnosis. However, the combination of low β-amyloid and high tau is reasonably specific for AD. The combination assay is commercially marketed and a positive test result may be of some value in differential diagnosis. However, the high false-negative rate limits its routine clinical applicability.

Assays for neural thread protein (NTP) have also been developed for commercial applications. NTP is a neuronal cytoskeletal component expressed in neuritic plaques. NTP can be detected in CSF and urine, but its value in diagnosis is controversial. As with other proposed biomarkers for AD, key questions related to the assays' positive and negative predictive values in mild cases remain unanswered in the literature. In addition, the specificity of the purported relationship between CSF neural thread protein and the pathophysiology of AD has been questioned.[22] Despite intensive marketing to both practitioners and patients, this assay is not in general clinical use as of 2003.

Approaches to Implementing Supplemental Tests

Clinical diagnosis through the use of validated criteria and practice guidelines, like those presented in Chapters 4 and 5, remains the best way to define and differentiate the various causes of dementia. When the clinical criteria cannot be met, or when diagnostic certainty is low, referral is indicated. For a generalist, the most appropriate referral would be to a specialist, such as a geriatrician, a neurologist, or a psychiatrist specializing in geriatrics or neuropsychiatry. Even among specialists, clinical referrals may be more useful than technological approaches. In medical schools, for example, neurologists with subspecialty training in dementia, geriatric neurology, or behavioral neurology may be available as a resource for patients and families. Their expertise lies in differential diagnosis and appropriate therapeutic options. For questions of psychotropic drug management, a neuropsychiatrist or geriatric psychiatrist can be of great value. In addition, many large hospitals operate interdisciplinary dementia assessment programs that can guide appropriate use of the expensive, and frequently noninformative, studies outlined in this chapter. These comprehensive programs can also provide a second opinion, manage family issues, and outline therapeutic options. Neuropsychology evaluation can also be considered a clinical specialty referral, especially useful in teasing out subtle patterns of impairment that clarify difficult differential diagnoses.

When clinical referral is not an option, further anatomic imaging may be appropriate. As noted, any patient who has cognitive symptoms associated with focal neurologic symptoms or signs, such as unilateral weakness (hemiparesis), diplopia, or Babinski's sign, warrants imaging. MRI is likely to be most informative in such individuals. When the dementia is not associated with focal findings but there are concerns about an atypical course or an unusual cognitive/behavioral pattern, CT is likely to be adequate. When dementia is advanced and the clinician is being asked questions of practical management rather than diagnosis—such as appropriateness for nursing home placement or optimal medications for behavioral control—the value of imaging is low.

If a clinical syndrome of dementia is present but the presentation is ambiguous or the clinical diagnostic certainty is low, tests of brain function, such as SPECT or EEG, may provide useful information. SPECT can provide important clues to the functional anatomy of the disease and clarify the clinical relevance of stroke or depression in a patient with mixed findings. For instance, the patient with multiple vasculopathic risk factors, memory dysfunction, and a prominent dysexecutive state on cognitive examination, no focal signs on neurologic examination, and nonspecific MRI findings, might have AD (most likely), mixed dementia, a 'pure' VaD, depression, or a form of frontal dementia. The pattern of hypoperfusion on SPECT can help clarify between these possibilities. Similarly, EEG is most useful when there is strong consideration of metabolic contributors to cognitive dysfunction, or the course suggests Creutzfeldt-Jakob disease. Therefore, in patients for whom there is suspicion for one of these conditions, or who do not meet clinical criteria for one of the common degenerative illnesses, EEG may be indicated.

Genetic testing has not been established to provide any major advantages over careful clinical diagnosis and the recommended approaches to demented patients. It may be useful to establish the exact genetic cause in some families with autosomal-dominant early-onset AD, but a negative test in an affected person does not change the heritable risk since there remain undiscovered mutations associated with familial disease. Similarly, the diagnostic advantages of AD-specific CSF and urinary assays remain to be demonstrated.

In summary, the decision to use supplemental testing should be dictated by the degree of diagnostic certainty after a well-considered approach to clinical diagnosis. The implications for the practical application of the results, whether positive or negative, should be clear before testing is ordered. If the result is unlikely to alter treatment or prognosis, the indication for the testing is low. In the future, as more sensitive and specific testing procedures are developed, such tests may play a much more important role, especially in mild phases of common dementing illnesses.

References

1.   American Academy of Neurology: Practice parameters for diagnosis and evaluation of dementia (summary statement): report of the Quality Standards Subcommittee of the American Academy of Neurology. *Neurology* 1994;44:2203-2206.

2.   Alexander EM, Wagner EH, Buchner DM, et al: Do surgical brain lesions present as isolated dementia? A population-based study. *J Am Geriatr Soc* 1995;43:138-143.

3.   Hachinski VC, Potter P, Merskey H: Leuko-araiosis. *Arch Neurol* 1987;44:21-23.

4.   Goto K, Ishii N, Fukasawa H: Diffuse white-matter disease in the geriatric population: a clinical, neuropathological, and CT study. *Radiology* 1981;141:687-695.

5.   Hendrie HC, Farlow MR, Austrom MG, et al: Foci of increased T2 signal intensity on brain MR scans of healthy elderly subjects. *Am J Neuroradiol* 1989;10:703-707.

6.   Giacometti AR, Davis PC, Alazraki NP, et al: Anatomic and physiologic imaging of Alzheimer's disease. In: Friedland RP, ed. Alzheimer's disease update. *Clin Geriatr Med* 1994;10:277-298.

7.   Ritchie K: Neuropsychological assessment in Alzheimer's disease: Current status and future directions. *Int Psychogeriatr* 1997;9(suppl 1):95-104.

8.   Ryan JJ, Paolo AM, Oehlert ME: Dementia screening: A tale of two tests. *VA Pract* 1989;6:51-54.

9.   Niederehe G: Depression and memory impairment in the aged. In: Poon LW, ed. *Handbook for Clinical Memory Assessment in Older Adults*. Washington, DC, American Psychological Association, 1986, pp 226-237.

10.   Shimomura T, Mori E, Yamashita H, et al: Cognitive loss in dementia with Lewy bodies and Alzheimer's disease. *Arch Neurol* 1998;55:1547-1552.

11.   Jobst KA, Hindley NJ, King E, et al: The diagnosis of Alzheimer's disease: a question of image? *J Clin Psychiatry* 1994;55 (suppl):22-31.

12.   Claus JJ, Vanharskamp F, Breteler MM, et al: The diagnostic value of SPECT with Tc 99m HMPAO in Alzheimer's disease: a population-based study. *Neurology* 1994;44:454-461.

13. Newberg AB, Alavi A, Payner F: Single photon emission computed tomography in Alzheimer's disease and related disorders. *Neuroimaging Clin North Am* 1995;5:103-123.

14. Mentis MJ, Horwitz B, Grady CL, et al: Visual cortical dysfunction in Alzheimer's disease evaluated with a temporally graded "stress test" during PET. *Am J Psychiatry* 1996;153:32-40.

15. Robinson DJ, Merskey H, Blume WT, et al: Electroencephalography as an aid in the exclusion of Alzheimer's disease. *Arch Neurol* 1994;51:280-284.

16. Rosen I: Electroencephalography as a diagnostic tool in dementia. *Dementia Geriatr Cogn Disord* 1997;8:110-116.

17. Claus JJ, Strijers RL, Jonkman EJ, et al: The diagnostic value of electroencephalography in mild senile dementia. *Clin Neurophysiol* 1999;110:825-832.

18. Mayeux R, Saunders AM, Shea S, et al: Utility of the apolipoprotein E genotype in the diagnosis of Alzheimer's disease. Alzheimer's Disease Centers Consortium on Apolipoprotein E and Alzheimer's Disease. *N Engl J Med* 1998;338:506-511.

19. Kawanishi C, Suzuki K, Odawara T, et al: Neuropathological evaluation and apolipoprotein E gene polymorphism analysis in diffuse Lewy body disease. *J Neurol Sci* 1996;136:140-142.

20. Tamaoka A, Sawamura N, Fukushima T, et al: Amyloid beta protein 42(43) in cerebrospinal fluid of patients with Alzheimer's disease. *J Neurol Sci* 1997;148:41-45.

21. Arai H, Terajima M, Miura M, et al: Tau in cerebrospinal fluid: a potential diagnostic marker in Alzheimer's disease. *Ann Neurol* 1995;38:649-652.

22. Blennow K, Wallin A, Chong JK: Cerebrospinal fluid 'neuronal thread protein' comes from serum by passage over the blood-brain barrier. *Neurodegeneration* 1995;4:187-193.

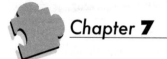

Chapter **7**

Models of Pharmacotherapy in AD

For many years, Alzheimer's disease (AD) was considered an untreatable disorder. This was a fallacy, since dementia has always been treatable with psychosocial interventions. Family-based education and intervention remain the cornerstones of therapy, but treatment options have expanded since useful AD-specific drug therapies emerged in the 1990s.

The pathologic processes of AD remain irreversible and incurable, but this does not imply that the clinical syndrome of AD cannot be modified. Pharmacotherapy is a useful tool in the management of the primary symptom complex in people with AD, namely progressive cognitive decline resulting in the loss of function in everyday life. This chapter outlines principles and specifics of drug therapy to treat the progressive loss of cognition and daily functioning caused by AD. Chapter 8 examines the specifics of cholinesterase inhibitor therapy in Alzheimer's disease. Approaches to difficult behaviors are covered in Chapter 9, and the complex issues of interdisciplinary and psychosocial disease state management are addressed in Chapter 10.

Potential Treatment Models

An essential point in treatment of AD is the recognition that, if left untreated, it is an inexorably progressive, debilitating, terminal illness. Therefore, any treatment that

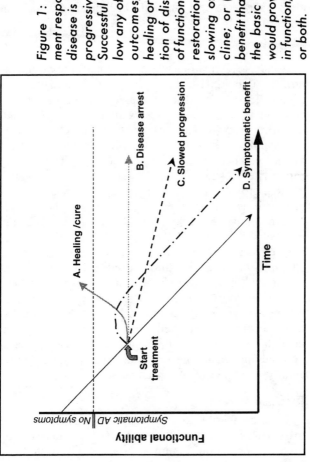

Figure 1: Models of treatment response. Alzheimer's disease is characterized by progressive loss of function. Successful therapy might follow any of several possible outcomes, including: (A) healing or cure, with resolution of disability; (B) arrest of functional decline without restoration of function; (C) slowing of the rate of decline; or (D) symptomatic benefit that, without altering the basic disease process, would provide improvement in function, delay in decline, or both.

reduces or delays progression, even if it does not lead to clinically evident improvement, provides a valuable benefit to the patient.

Because research advances in AD are moving rapidly, it is important for the potential prescriber of any AD therapy to have a clear understanding of how a new drug might fit into a treatment model. Several potential models for therapy to treat functional decline are illustrated in Figure 1.

Healing or Cure

An ideal AD treatment would restore function and return the individual to his or her presymptomatic state (Figure 1, curve A.) This is impractical because of several factors, including the observation that cell death and degeneration are probably present for years before the earliest symptom of AD emerges. Despite excitement about the development of viable neuronal cells in adults,[1] the carefully orchestrated system that regulates neuronal migration, growth, and synapse formation during embryogenesis is not known to be operational in the healthy senescent human, much less the AD brain. Therefore, any new cells that form are likely to be 'all dressed up with nowhere to go.' Furthermore, other evidence suggests that attempts at regeneration through cell division may be fatal for adult neurons.[2] Neuronal implantation strategies, such as those tried in Parkinson's disease, are plagued because neuronal degeneration in AD is widespread rather than being restricted to well-defined nuclei. Fundamental breakthroughs in the basic science of neuronal regeneration and functional synapse formation are required before curative therapies for AD become viable.

Disease Arrest

If it is not feasible to permanently restore the functional loss, then perhaps the next best approach would be to stop disease progression (Figure 1, curve B). Given the state of knowledge about AD pathophysiology, this may become a viable therapeutic option in the first decades of the 21st century, at least for some subtypes of AD. This approach requires a complete interruption of the pathophysiologic cascade that leads to synaptic withdrawal, neuronal dysfunction, and cell death.

Disease-arresting therapies may also help prevent the clinical expression of AD. If accurate, presymptomatic diagnosis for AD can be developed, clinicians could use disease-arresting therapies before functional disability appears. If the disease-arresting therapy was safe and inexpensive, it could become possible to institute population-based prevention, through inoculation (as was done for polio) or oral supplementation (as with public water fluoridation for dental caries). A sufficiently safe and cheap treatment would bypass the need for presymptomatic disease identification. From a public health perspective, presymptomatic disease arrest with population-wide implementation would be tantamount to curing AD within one generation.

Slowed Progression

Some treatments might not completely arrest the disease, but would still slow synaptic loss and neuronal death. This would alter the trajectory of decline (Figure 1, curve C). In some cases, these treatments might interfere with an early pathophysiologic event in AD, such as preventing the formation of insoluble amyloid fibrils in the brain. Alternatively, this kind of therapy could partially block the effect of AD pathophysiology on the neuron, making it more resistant to the triggers of cell death. For example, many practitioners began to prescribe vitamin E during the late 1990s because of the putative role of amyloid-induced oxidative damage to neuronal membranes. Vitamin E use is described in more detail later in this chapter.

Because the rate of neuronal loss is reduced, disease-slowing therapies should be associated with an increas-

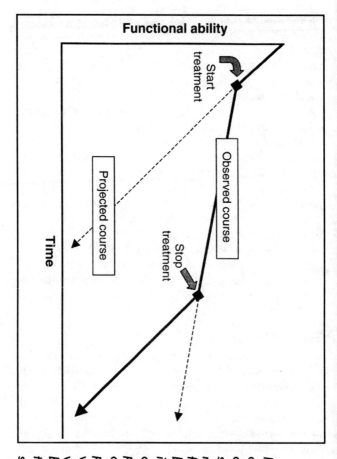

Figure 2: Effect of a disease-slowing agent. If a drug can slow decline, it would reduce the rate of functional loss caused by AD. When the drug is stopped, the rate of decline would be expected to return to the original slope. Longer periods of therapy would be associated with greater relative benefit, even though the treated patient is still worsening.

ing magnitude of benefit, relative to the untreated baseline, with longer duration of therapy. This does not mean that there will be no decline. It can be difficult to communicate to patients and families the concept that, even with 'effective' treatment, progressive functional loss is anticipated. Assessment of efficacy is troublesome because: (1) rates of decline are difficult to determine in clinical settings; (2) there are no effective surrogate markers of cell death; and (3) natural variations in decline exist within and across patients. If a therapy that has stopped or slowed decline is discontinued, the rate of decline would be expected to return to a course parallel to the projected, untreated course (Figure 2).

Symptomatic Benefit

Clinically, Alzheimer's disease can be summarized as a progressive loss of function over time. Therefore, it is possible to reduce the symptomatic expression of AD without altering the fundamental pathophysiologic processes that contribute to cell death. Unlike the treatment models described above, symptomatic therapy is designed to maximize neuronal function (ie, transsynaptic communication) without affecting the rate of neuronal loss. This approach to treatment is associated with 2 therapeutic goals: (1) improvement in function, and (2) delay in decline (Figure 1, curve D). Since the rate of neuronal death is relatively unaffected, once decline is again evident, it should proceed at the same pace as the untreated course. The advantage to the patient on this type of therapy is the prolonged ability at, or perhaps above, the level of function where treatment begins. Decline occurs later in life, increasing the likelihood of death from other age-related causes at a higher level of function. When symptomatic therapy is discontinued, a rapid drop in abilities is anticipated, bringing patients back to the functional level where they would have been without treatment (Figure 3).

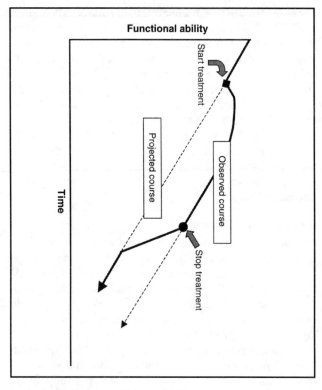

Figure 3: Effects of symptomatic therapy. Response to an agent providing symptomatic benefit without altering the underlying disease process can be expected to include improvement or stabilization of symptoms for a period of time. As the disease process worsens, functional decline resumes but at a later point in time. When treatment is stopped, a rapid loss of function can occur as the treated patient returns to the course of expected progression without treatment. This rapid drop in function can be used to ascertain that treatment had been benefiting the patient, and is frequently an indication to resume therapy.

Assessing Therapeutic Outcome

A major challenge in AD therapeutics is assessing the outcome of treatment. Unlike hypertension or diabetes mellitus, in which objective numbers are used to determine the effectiveness of therapy, AD treatment response in clinical practice depends primarily on subjective assessment.

It is important to remember, however, that the long-term goal of antihypertensive therapy is not to lower the number on the sphygmomanometer, but rather to prevent the complications of chronic hypertension. In the same way, it is not the goal of AD therapy simply to raise the score on a mental status examination, but rather to reduce the individual's disability or prevent its worsening, to the greatest extent possible. Continuing the hypertension model, this approach can be viewed as identical to measuring successful antihypertensive treatment outcomes as reduced incidence of myocardial infarction and stroke.

Other factors that complicate assessment include limited insight and motivation in the AD patient. Vital outcome information must, therefore, be obtained from surrogates, most often family members in a caregiving role. Even 'objective' measures of cognition, like the Mini-Mental State Examination (MMSE), depend on the patient's motivation to comply with testing, understanding of the task demands, and ability to organize voluntary responses.

These challenges deter some physicians from ever prescribing drug treatment in AD patients. However, several drugs have received regulatory approval for treatment of AD (see Chapter 8), and more are on the way, so the practitioner who chooses not to prescribe must consider the potential legal consequences of falling below an emerging standard of care.

Assessment Domains

Therapeutic outcomes in AD are often classified into 3 major domains: (1) cognition, (2) behavior, and (3) daily

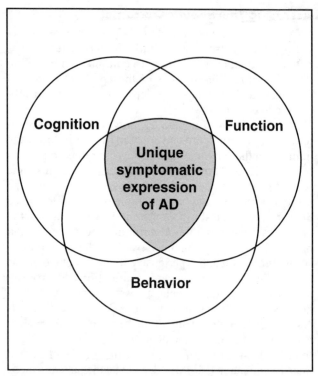

Figure 4: Assessment domains. When assessing the effectiveness of therapy, cognitive, behavioral, and functional domains (ie, activities of daily living) should be considered in light of the patient's individual symptom pattern.

function. These categories are artifactual, being based on the intent of the instruments used to measure them in research settings. Each individual affected by the disease will have a unique overlap of symptoms in these 3 realms, without clear boundaries between them. In addition, these domains exist in the context of a lifetime of individual development. Personal background, such as age, education, personality, life experience, social support, and concurrent illnesses, will affect an individual's response to AD in these aspects of life (Figure 4). It should, therefore, be clear that no single measure can be used to accurately assess treatment outcome across all individuals, or even within one person throughout the disease course. The choice of outcome measures will depend on the baseline behavioral and cognitive style of the patient, the individual character of the symptoms, the properties of the chosen drugs, and—perhaps most importantly—the priorities of the patient and the caregiver. If the primary goal of the caregiver is reduced sleep disturbance, then therapies targeted at improving memory performance are likely to be deemed unsuccessful. This would be akin to choosing an antiarrhythmic to treat hypertension.

Cognition

In clinical trials, cognitive response to treatment is usually measured on standardized tests like the MMSE to measure treatment response. However, there are drawbacks to using the MMSE in practice. The test is heavily weighted toward memory and orientation, but these areas may not respond to the treatment class of medication being used. It is, therefore, important to choose outcome measures that best reflect the properties of the treatment being employed. For example, acetylcholinesterase inhibitors are the mainstays of symptomatic therapy for AD, and research suggests that attention abilities show the greatest response to cholinergic manipulation.[3] Attention-demanding tests, such as serial subtraction, or reciting the months in reverse order, might therefore be predicted to be more efficient measures of response to this type of therapy.

The caregiver's report on cognitive abilities cannot be discounted. The demands on cognition in the 'real world' are far more intricate than tests the clinician can present and measure in the office. Therefore, the caregiver may be able to report cognitive improvement that falls below the threshold of bedside testing. Caregivers might report that the patient seems brighter, sharper, or better able to understand conversation. In the end, the caregiver's assessment provides the ecological validity of the response. Even a normalization of the MMSE to 30 out of 30 is unimportant if no change in day-to-day cognitive ability is noted outside the office. This is also important when assessing non-AD forms of dementia, especially frontal dementia, which may not impair MMSE performance in its early stages.

Behavior

Behavior change in AD is ubiquitous. Some behavior changes reflect loss of normal function, similar to the loss of normal cognition. These include self-centeredness (loss of empathy), apathy (loss of motivation), and anosognosia (loss of insight into ability). There are no easily administered bedside instruments to measure these behaviors. It is, therefore, imperative to elicit caregiver assessment of these symptoms. With successful treatment, a caregiver might report that the patient is more emotionally responsive and affectionate. Improved motivation can be reflected in improved levels of activity or less resistance to self-care, such as bathing. Improved insight can be an adverse experience in some people, who become distressed when they recognize the degree of their impairments. Generally, this is unusual with treatments, and the risk for deleterious insight should not deter a clinician from prescribing a therapy that may otherwise lead to improvement.

Many adverse behaviors seen in AD represent abnormal, unwanted additions to the behavioral repertoire. Outside the context of dementia, these occur most commonly in delirium and primary psychiatric syndromes. They include delusions, hallucinations, and depression. Agitation is frequently described in AD patients and probably represents a nonspecific effect of cognitive and behavioral control deficits. The general pharmacologic approach to these syndromes as they complicate dementia is addressed in Chapter 9.

Function

Since dementia is defined on the basis of functional loss, assessment of this realm is essential in determining treatment outcome. In practice, function can be divided into instrumental activities, like driving, managing household finances, cooking, etc, and basic activities that include bathing, feeding, and personal hygiene. Taken together, these abilities constitute activities of daily living (ADL). Unfortunately, most instruments designed to assess ADL are either too cumbersome for office use or insensitive to the magnitude of improvement that results from available therapies. Documenting functional level with instruments such as the FAQ or PSMS (Chapter 5) is perhaps most useful for assessing the rate of decline for disease-slowing or -delaying treatments.

Other Therapeutic Outcomes

A frequent correlate of functional ability is quality of life (QOL). Many instruments have been proposed to assess QOL, but they generally have limited use in routine clinical practice, and are not well suited for the specific problems of AD. Since AD patients frequently lack insight, they may not perceive a change in their QOL, but family members in a caregiving role often report that their own QOL suffers as a direct result of their loved one's AD. Improvements in patient cognition, behavior, or function that fall below the threshold of effective office measurement may nonetheless result in improved caregiver QOL. Therefore, caregiver reports about their QOL present another target area for monitoring patient treatment response.

When improvement in ability is not detected, families may seek reassurance that the therapy is delaying symptom progression. In many cases, the clinician will attempt to assess the rate of progression in comparison to an unobserved period of progression before treatment. Because of wide individual variation in the rates of decline between persons with AD and even over time within individuals, there are no useful instruments for assessing rate of progression in routine clinical settings.

There are also economic incentives for delaying decline. Preventing MMSE decline in a moderately impaired patient can result in total health-care cost reductions in the range of $750 to $2,500 annually.[4] Another study in a managed-care organization model suggested that drug intervention actually reduced other medical costs per AD patient, but that the cost reduction did not completely offset the price of the medication.[5]

Cholinergic Therapy

An important model for cognitive dysfunction in AD is the cholinergic hypothesis. AD is characterized by extensive cell loss in the basal nuclei of the forebrain, including the nucleus basalis of Meynert. These basal forebrain nuclei house the cell bodies of neurons that produce the neurotransmitter acetylcholine (ACh). Axons from these cells synapse throughout the cerebral cortex, especially the frontal lobe, and also project to hippocampal structures. These regions are vital to attention, learning, and memory. Many studies show reduced levels of cerebral cortical ACh function in AD, and the degree of reduction correlates with the amount of cognitive impairment. Supplementing cortical ACh has, therefore, been an important goal in AD drug development. Three distinct approaches to boosting cortical ACh synaptic function have been developed for use in AD. These are: (1) supplement production of ACh, (2) activate ACh receptors with a pharmacologic agonist, or (3) inhibit destruction of naturally produced ACh.

Supplementing Production

One approach to supplementing the production of ACh is to maximize the substrates available for the synthetic reaction. Precursor supplementation is a well-understood model of therapy in other neurodegenerative syndromes, such as Parkinson's disease (PD). In PD, levodopa, a precursor to dopamine, is administered to enhance dopamine synthesis in the surviving pool of substantia nigra neurons.

ACh is produced at axon terminals by the action of cholineacetyltransferase (CAT) on acetyl-CoA and choline, releasing CoA to be reused. Acetyl-CoA is produced intracellularly and is not amenable to direct pharmacologic manipulation. However, choline can enter the brain from the bloodstream. Therefore, both choline and its precursor phosphatidylcholine (lecithin) have been administered to AD patients. Unfortunately, despite raising blood levels of choline, these agents have no consistently observable clinical effect on function or cognition.[6,7] Nonetheless, this model of therapy is still promoted among some enthusiasts of alternative medicine, and both choline and lecithin are easily available in health food stores.

Agonist Therapy

Like all classic neurotransmitters, acetylcholine operates on cells via receptors. The brain contains both muscarinic and nicotinic classes of ACh receptors. Immense challenges exist to developing selective ACh agonists to treat AD. One problem with agonist therapy is that systemically administered drugs often affect not only brain ACh receptors, but also cholinergic receptors throughout the body, including the autonomic nervous system and neuromuscular junctions. The drugs can create uncomfortable (hypersalivation) or dangerous (cardiac arrhythmia) side effects.

In the brain, ACh receptors are distributed on both presynaptic and postsynaptic cells. There is a complex cholinergic chemistry involving multiple receptor types, associated with different time-courses of action and second messengers. An ideal cholinergic agonist would have to replicate as closely as possible the effects of endogenous

ACh at the synapse. However, to minimize systemic effects, most agonists developed for AD therapy are selectively active at only a subset of ACh receptors. This truncates the overall response and may render the treatment less effective.

Finally, brain cholinergic transmission is an on-demand (phasic) phenomenon. ACh is released only when an action potential reaches the presynaptic nerve terminal. In contrast, agonist agents would be active at some constant (tonic) level related to synaptic concentration of the drug. The future of cholinergic agonist therapies in AD is unclear because of their limited ability to replicate the dynamic interplay between neurotransmitter release, postsynaptic response, and presynaptic regulation.

Agonist Clinical Trials

As of 2003, no agonists have been approved for AD therapy in the United States. Despite the challenges to developing this class of drugs, several agents have undergone large-scale clinical testing in AD patients. Xanomeline is a selective activator of the postsynaptic M1 muscarinic agonist. It shows some efficacy in improving cognition and behavioral disorders in AD, but has a high rate of side effects that led more than half the patients taking effective doses to discontinue treatment.[8,9]

Nicotine is an agonist at nicotinic receptors in the central nervous system (CNS). Acute injections and chronic administration of nicotine result in memory enhancement,[10] but the clinical relevance of such improvements has been questioned.[11] More highly selective nicotinic agonists have been developed with the hope of achieving cognitive improvement with reduced risk for systemic side effects. Preliminary testing of these agents is promising.[12]

Inhibiting ACh Degradation

Acetylcholine is hydrolyzed into acetate and choline by the intrasynaptic enzyme acetylcholinesterase (AChE).

AChE is one of the most efficient enzymes to be characterized. A single AChE molecule can hydrolyze 5,000 ACh molecules per second.[13] Inhibiting AChE at the neuromuscular junction is a primary model of therapy for myasthenia gravis. In myasthenia, there is an immune-mediated reduction in postsynaptic ACh receptors. In contrast, AD is characterized by a reduction of synaptic ACh release. In both cases, AChE inhibition prolongs the availability of the transmitter to the postsynaptic receptor. Antimyasthenia treatments depend on chemical structures that do not cross the blood-brain barrier to minimize CNS effects, but agents that enter the brain have the potential for neuromuscular effects. There are several subforms of AChE, as well as a closely related cholinesterase (butyrylcholinesterase) that is less specific to ACh. The pattern of activity these drugs exert across the different enzymes contributes significantly to both the efficacy and toxicity of AChE inhibition. Cholinesterase inhibitors are the mainstay of AD therapy. These agents are examined in more detail in Chapter 8.

Therapies to Slow Alzheimer's Disease Progression

As noted in Chapter 2, a cascade of events leads to cell death in AD. An extensive research effort exists dedicated to identifying potential targets for drug therapy that might interrupt this cascade. These targets include interfering with the production and deposition of insoluble amyloid, interrupting the microglial inflammatory response to amyloid, protecting the neuron against inflammatory products generated by the cascade, and supporting the ability of the neuron to resist damage (ie, neurotrophism).

Anti-Inflammatory Drugs

Epidemiologic studies suggest that regular use of non-steroidal anti-inflammatory drugs (NSAIDs) reduces the risk of Alzheimer's disease.[14] One preliminary 6-month trial of the NSAID indomethacin also suggests a disease-slowing effect for this agent, but widespread use of indomethacin is not indicated because of poor tolerability.[15] NSAIDs vary widely in their ability to cross the blood barrier, so the ability to generalize this finding to other drugs is poor. A much larger trial recently assessed the effect of prednisone, a potent steroidal anti-inflammatory agent, and found no effect for slowing AD progression over 1 year.[16] Large-scale, pharmaceutical industry and federally sponsored trials of nonselective NSAIDs and selective cyclo-oxygenase-2 inhibitors have reported preliminary results that are not promising. Much of the conceptual basis of these studies assumes a vital role for the cyclo-oxygenase pathways of inflammation in AD, but laboratory evidence suggests that other mediators of inflammation may be more important.[17]

Antioxidants

Despite the uncertainty of how amyloid triggers the production of neurotoxic inflammatory products, one outcome of the cascade appears to be free radical species that act to damage neuronal membranes. The best evidence for the protective effect of antioxidants in AD comes from a large-scale, double-blind, placebo-controlled study trial of the antioxidants high-dose vitamin E (α-tocopherol 2,000 IU daily) and selegiline (10 mg daily) in patients with moderate AD.[18] As appropriate for trials assessing effects on progression, cognitive improvement was not the outcome of interest. Instead, clinically relevant outcomes, such as nursing home placement, loss of daily functional abilities, and death, were observed. The results indicated that patients taking vitamin E, selegiline, or both reached these endpoints later than patients on placebo. There was no added value of combined treatment (Figure 5). Since the agents were equally effective alone or in combination, the better safety and lower cost for vitamin E suggests that it can be effective in slow-

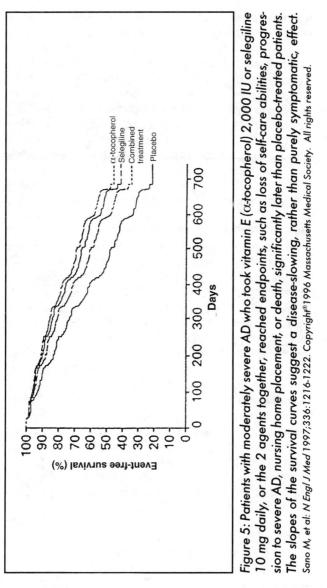

Figure 5: Patients with moderately severe AD who took vitamin E (α-tocopherol) 2,000 IU or selegiline 10 mg daily, or the 2 agents together, reached endpoints, such as loss of self-care abilities, progression to severe AD, nursing home placement, or death, significantly later than placebo-treated patients. The slopes of the survival curves suggest a disease-slowing, rather than purely symptomatic, effect.

ing AD progression. There has been concern among clinicians about the high dose of vitamin E, but in both the study and in clinical experience, 2,000 IU daily is well tolerated by nearly all patients. No reports to date assess the efficacy of lower (or higher) doses in comparison to the 2,000 IU dosage. Large-scale studies of α-tocopherol efficacy in earlier or later AD have not been reported to date. There is a federally sponsored multicenter trial assessing the effectiveness of vitamin E for preventing the transition from mild cognitive impairment to the full early-AD syndrome. While there are significant problems with overgeneralizing the results, many AD experts routinely advise high-dose vitamin E therapy, usually 800 to 1,000 IU b.i.d.

Neurotrophic Approaches

Since neuronal death leads to the symptoms of AD, neuronal growth factors have been hypothesized to offset the effects of toxic products on the cells. Many potential neurotrophic agents are peptides that cannot be taken orally because they are digested as proteins in the stomach. Therefore, alternative routes of administration are necessary. Nerve growth factor (NGF) has been instilled into the cerebral ventricles to test this hypothesis, but the degree of invasiveness and serious adverse effects prevent large-scale testing. More promising approaches, including intranasal absorption of peptides, are under study.

Estrogen is a steroidal hormone that has positive neurotrophic effects. Epidemiologic studies indicate that women who take estrogen replacement therapy after menopause may have a reduced risk of AD. This led to a double-blind, placebo-controlled study of estrogen replacement in women with AD, but no benefit was identified for the estrogen-treated group.[19]

Other Agents

A wide variety of other agents claim to affect AD progression. None are approved by the FDA for use in AD.

Many of these are marketed as nutritional supplements through direct advertising and health food stores. Few have been subjected to the standards of double-blind, placebo-controlled studies, so their efficacy claims are unestablished. Ginkgo biloba is a plant extract that is often asserted to have beneficial effects on memory. More recent studies appear to indicate that ginkgo has no direct beneficial effect on memory or cognition.[20] In one double-blind, placebo-controlled trial in patients with dementia, it had only minimal effects over a 1-year trial.[21] Many methodologic flaws limit the interpretation of these findings, but more recently, the United States government funded a very large, multicenter, double-blind, placebo-controlled trial of ginkgo. Results of this trial are not expected until 2004 or later.

Conclusions

Strong evidence supports the role of pharmacologic therapy in AD, particularly for patients in the mild and moderate stages. Effective therapy can promote and maintain cognition, behavior, and function, potentially leading to improvements in the quality of life for the patient and the caregiver. There may also be positive economic outcomes from well-considered therapeutic approaches. Most patients with mild or moderate AD can be predicted to show benefits from combined symptomatic therapy with a cholinesterase inhibitor and disease-slowing therapy with vitamin E. Setting appropriate expectations, both for the prescriber and for the family, is a vital part of successful intervention.

References

1. Eriksson PS, Perfilieva E, Bjork-Eriksson T, et al: Neurogenesis in the adult human hippocampus. *Nat Med* 1998;4:1313-1317.

2. Busser J, Geldmacher DS, Herrup K: Ectopic cell cycle proteins predict the sites of neuronal cell death in Alzheimer's disease brain. *J Neurosci* 1998;18:2801-2807.

3. Sahakian BJ, Coull JT: Tetrahydroaminoacridine (THA) in Alzheimer's disease: an assessment of attentional and mnemonic function using CANTAB. *Acta Neurol Scand Suppl* 1993; 149: 29-35.

4. Ernst RL, Hay JW, Fenn C, et al: Cognitive function and the costs of Alzheimer's disease. An exploratory study. *Arch Neurol* 1997;54:687-693.

5. Fillit H, Gutterman EM, Lewis B: Donepezil use in managed Medicare: effect on health care costs and utilization. *Clin Ther* 1999;21:2173-2185.

6. Thal LJ, Rosen W, Sharpless NS, et al: Choline chloride fails to improve cognition of Alzheimer's disease. *Neurobiol Aging* 1981;2:205-208.

7. Little A, Levy R, Chuaqui-Kidd P, et al: A double-blind, placebo-controlled trial of high-dose lecithin in Alzheimer's disease. *J Neurol Neurosurg Psychiatry* 1985;48:736-742.

8. Veroff AE, Bodick NC, Offen WW, et al: Efficacy of xanomeline in Alzheimer disease: cognitive improvement measured using the Computerized Neuropsychological Test Battery (CNTB). *Alzheimer Dis Assoc Disord* 1998;12:304-312.

9. Bodick NC, Offen WW, Levey AI, et al: Effects of xanomeline, a selective muscarinic receptor agonist, on cognitive function and behavioral symptoms in Alzheimer's disease. *Arch Neurol* 1997;54:465-473.

10. White HK, Levin ED: Four-week nicotine skin patch treatment effects on cognitive performance in Alzheimer's disease. *Psychopharmacology* 1999;143:158-165.

11. Snaedal J, Johannesson T, Jonsson JE, et al: The effects of nicotine in dermal plaster on cognitive functions in patients with Alzheimer's disease. *Dementia* 1996;7:47-52.

12. Potter A, Corwin J, Lang J, et al: Acute effects of the selective cholinergic channel activator (nicotinic agonist) ABT-418 in Alzheimer's disease. *Psychopharmacology* 1999;142: 334-342.

13. Cooper JR, Bloom FE, Roth RH: *The Biochemical Basis of Neuropharmacology*, 6th ed. New York, Oxford University Press, 1991, pp 190-219.

14. McGeer PL, Schulzer M, McGeer EG: Arthritis and anti-inflammatory agents as possible protective factors for Alzheimer's

disease: a review of 17 epidemiologic studies. *Neurology* 1996;47: 425-432.

15. Rogers J, Kirby LC, Hempelman SR, et al: Clinical trial of indomethacin in Alzheimer's disease. *Neurology* 1993;43:1609-1611.

16. Aisen PS, Davis KL, Berg JD, et al: A randomized controlled trial of prednisone in Alzheimer's disease. Alzheimer's Disease Cooperative Study. *Neurology* 2000;54:588-593.

17. Combs CK, Johnson DE, Karlo JC, et al: Inflammatory mechanisms in Alzheimer's disease: inhibition of β-amyloid-stimulated proinflammatory responses and neurotoxicity by PPARγ agonists. *J Neurosci* 2000;20:558-567.

18. Sano M, Ernesto C, Thomas RG, et al: A controlled trial of selegiline, α-tocopherol, or both as treatment for Alzheimer's disease. The Alzheimer's Disease Cooperative Study. *N Engl J Med* 1997;336:1216-1222.

19. Mulnard RA, Cotman CW, Kawas C, et al: Estrogen replacement therapy for treatment of mild to moderate Alzheimer disease: a randomized controlled trial. Alzheimer's Disease Cooperative Study. *JAMA* 2000;283:1007-1015.

20. Solomon PR, Adams F, Silver A, et al: Ginkgo for memory enhancement: a randomized controlled trial. *JAMA* 2002;288 :835-840.

21. Le Bars PL, Katz MM, Berman N, et al: A placebo-controlled, double-blind, randomized trial of an extract of ginkgo biloba for dementia. North American EGb Study Group. *JAMA* 1997; 278:1327-1332.

Chapter **8**

Cholinesterase Inhibitor Therapy for Alzheimer's Disease

O f the various modes of action for symptomatic treatment of Alzheimer's disease (AD) reviewed in Chapter 7, only the acetylcholinesterase inhibitor (AChEI) class of drugs had demonstrated sufficient efficacy to gain marketing approval in the United States by 2003. The three approved agents most often used are donepezil (Aricept®), galantamine (Reminyl®), and rivastigmine (Exelon®). A fourth agent, tacrine (Cognex®), is used only occasionally because of hepatotoxicity problems. There remains considerable controversy over the clinical meaningfulness of the results reported for these drugs. Nonetheless, the American Academy of Neurology's evidence-based practice parameter for treatment of dementia recommends AChEIs as the standard of care for mild-to-moderate Alzheimer's disease.[1] This chapter reviews both the general approach with AChEIs and the specific efficacy data for each agent.

General Approach With AChEIs

Treatment initiation with AChEIs should be considered when AD is diagnosed. Convergent evidence suggests that delaying treatment can result in reduced benefit in cognitive ability compared to patients who start therapy earlier.[2,3] Despite marketing claims implying superior efficacy because of differences in mechanism of action, the pattern of efficacy is very similar among the approved agents (Table 1). For all three agents, the small mean improvements in cognition are achieved within 3 months of starting therapy, and a high proportion of patients maintain at least baseline levels of cognition for 6 to 12 months.[2-7] In contrast, the pharmacokinetic profiles of the three agents differ considerably[8] (Table 2). Nonetheless, ease of use and tolerability generally influence the choice of a specific drug for an individual AD patient more than efficacy or pharmacokinetic factors.

Managing Expectations

Patients, and especially their families, should be counseled about realistic expectations from AChEI therapy. Acetylcholinesterase inhibitors do not restore dead neurons or reverse the passage of time. Dramatic reversal of memory impairment is unlikely and families should be made aware that subtle but genuine improvements in attentiveness, apathy, and conversational language are more common than frank memory enhancement. For many families, the value ascribed to even these relatively small gains is more than sufficient to offset the cost of the drug and the risks for toxicity. Clinically meaningful restoration of activities of daily living (ADL) is rare. Nonetheless, preservation of daily function (ie, delaying decline or "holding one's own") remains a valuable goal. Persistent AChEI therapy is associated with significantly reduced risk for,[9,10] or delayed,[11] institutionalization (Figure 1). Although these are major goals for families coping with AD,[12] they may not be evident for years.

Time Course to Response

In clinical trials, cognitive test scores increase over 12 weeks of therapy (Figure 2).[2-7] The most common error in the prescription of AChEIs is to discontinue therapy when

Table 1: Efficacy of Cholinesterase Inhibitors in 6-month Trials

	Donepezil 5-10 mg/day
Mean ADAS-cog improvement	2.3-3.1
% of subjects improving >7 points on ADAS-cog	15%-26%
Active treatment subjects stable (ADAS-cog ≥ baseline) at 6 months	82%-83%
Placebo patients stable at 6 months	59%
Net proportion of subjects improved relative to placebo at 6 months	23%-24%

Table 2: Pharmacokinetics[8]

Characteristic	Donepezil
Mechanism of action	Selective acetylcholinesterase inhibition
Plasma half-life	50-70 h
Elimination pathway	Hepatic
Metabolism	CYP 2D6 CYP 3A4
Protein binding	96%
Doses/Day	1

Galantamine 16-32 mg/day	Rivastigmine 6-12 mg/day
3.4-4.0	1.7-4.4
15%-20%	12%-18%
58%-64%	55%-56%
40%-44%	27%-45%
20%-25%	10%-29%

Galantamine	Rivastigmine
Acetylcholinesterase inhibition + nicotinic modulatory receptor effect	Butyryl cholinesterase + acetylcholinesterase inhibition
5-7 h	0.6-2.0 h
Renal + hepatic	Renal
CYP 2D6 CYP 3A4	Cholinesterase-mediated hydrolysis
18%	40%
2	2

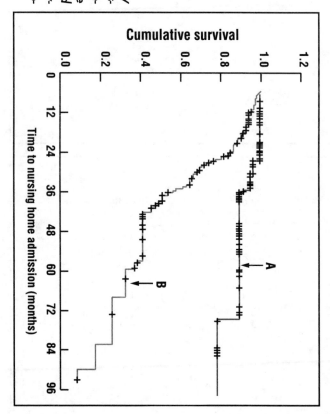

Figure 1: Persistent therapy with AChEI agents (A) was associated with significantly reduced risk for nursing home placement when compared with matched patients receiving no AChEI (B) in this retrospective study.[10]

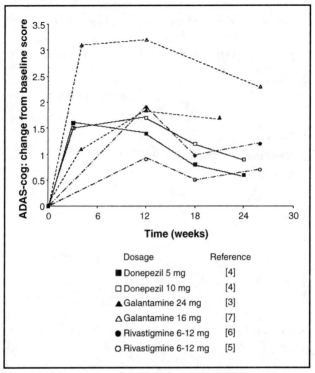

Figure 2: Time course of response to AChEIs at recommended doses. The magnitude of the effects can not be compared because of differences in the placebo response in each trial (see Table 1).

clear-cut improvements are not evident after a brief course of treatment, sometimes a month or less. When a decision is made to prescribe an AChE inhibitor, it is important to provide a full trial before discontinuing the drug. This process is similar to antidepressant use, another neurotransmitter-based treatment approach. Most clinicians are comfortable with the 6-week to 8-week delay to peak efficacy for antidepressants. A similar period, sometimes several

Table 3: Proportion of Patients With Common GI Side Effects Associated With AChEI Treatment (from package inserts)[14-16]

	Donepezil 5-10 mg (6-week titration)	
	Drug (%)	Placebo (%)
Nausea	5-6	6
Diarrhea	8-9	5
Vomiting	3-5	3
Anorexia	3	2
Weight loss	3	1

* Current recommendations suggest dose titration at not less than 4-week intervals. Longer intervals between

months, is necessary before efficacy or failure of cholinesterase inhibitors can be determined.

Safety

Three of the 4 AChEIs in use have been shown in clinical trials to be generally safe. Tacrine is no longer routinely used because it has a significant risk for hepatotoxicity not seen with the other AChEI agents. However, because of potentially dangerous, cholinergically mediated complications, these agents should be used cautiously in patients with asthma, gastric or peptic ulcers, chronic diarrhea, or bradycardia and/or bundle branch block.[13] But these conditions are not absolute contraindications to prescribing AChEIs. Galantamine may require dose adjustment or limitation with hepatic or renal failure.[14]

Galantamine (16-24 mg) (4-week titration)		Rivastigmine (6-12 mg) (1-week forced titration)*	
Drug (%)	Placebo (%)	Drug (%)	Placebo (%)
13-17	5	47	12
6-12	6	19	11
6-10	1	31	6
7-9	3	17	3
5	1	3	1

dose escalation have been associated with lower rates of adverse GI effects for AchEIs.[16]

Tolerability

Because acetylcholinesterase is the primary gastrointestinal (GI) motility-enhancing transmitter, nausea, anorexia, and diarrhea or loose stools should be anticipated. Not surprisingly, in the pivotal trials leading to FDA approval of these agents, GI side effects were most common (Table 3). Despite similarities in efficacy and safety, there are clinically appreciable differences among the three drugs in the frequency of these adverse events. The number of patients with GI side effects was highest with rivastigmine,[15] intermediate with galantamine,[14] and lowest with donepezil.[16] Gastrointestinal side effects are also the principal limiting factor in practice, but often at rates lower than those reported in clinical trials. Clinical experience also suggests that patients with a history of frequent digestive complaints may be more prone to recurrence of these with AChEI therapy. Slower dose titration appears to result in fewer adverse GI effects.[16] Dose reduction is warranted if these symptoms become intolerable to the patient. If the positive effect of treatment is such that the patient or family is unwilling to discontinue therapy or reduce dosing, peripherally acting atropine-like agents, such as glycopyrrolate (Robinul®) 1 mg q.d.- t.i.d., may be useful in reducing GI side effects.

Low frequencies of clinically significant weight loss ($\geq$ 7% of body weight at baseline) have been observed with all three drugs. However, rivastigmine's package insert carries a warning that high rates of weight loss have occurred at doses exceeding 9 mg/day (18% to 26% rivastigmine vs 4% to 6% placebo).[15] In contrast to rivastigmine's dose-related effect, weight loss associated with the increasing severity of illness does not seem to be magnified by AChEI treatment. The incidence of clinically significant weight loss was similar between donepezil-treated and placebo-treated patients in trials conducted in elderly nursing home AD patients (9% donepezil vs 6% placebo)[17] and in moderate to severe AD patients (7% donepezil vs 8% placebo).[18]

Other cholinergic adverse effects appear to be more idiosyncratic. These include sleep disturbance, vivid dreams, muscle cramps, increased oronasal secretions, urinary incontinence, and, rarely, agitation and delirium. A vagotonic bradycardia has been observed in some patients, but it is generally asymptomatic. When sleep disturbances occur, altering the dosing schedule may help alleviate them (eg, moving donepezil administration to the morning or the second dose of galantamine or rivastigmine to dinner time). No unique pattern of these less common symptoms has been identified for the AChEIs in use.

Drug Interactions

In the elderly population most at risk for dementia, polypharmacy is common and the addition of any drug may entail unpredictable problems. Fortunately, few clinically relevant interactions of AChEIs have been identified, and the overall incidence of events attributed to AChEIs interacting with other drugs is very low. Because AChEIs potentiate the effects of succinylcholine-type agents, some caution is warranted when surgery is planned. The anesthesiologist should be consulted in advance and a plan formulated for managing the AChEI. Brief withdrawal of the AChEI may be necessary, but this requires caution and a plan for reinstituting therapy at the earliest possible juncture.

Discontinuation

AChEIs have not demonstrated a major effect on neuronal survival. Patients can be expected to decline during prolonged treatment as neurons continue to die. The clinical trials experience strongly suggests, however, that a patient receiving treatment will likely have improved function compared to his or her projected condition, at the same point in time, if left untreated. This effect is observable for as long as 3 years. Therefore, decline in cognition or function from baseline levels is not, by itself, an indication for discontinuing therapy. Discontinuation of these drugs has been associated with rapid declines in cognitive test scores and global function, which become evident within weeks.

The primary indications for AChEI discontinuation are perceived lack of efficacy and intolerable side effects. Other factors can also influence the desire to discontinue therapy, including the cost of drug therapy, patient resistance to treatment, or other social factors. If the clinician or family decides that the treatment appears to be ineffective, a therapeutic withdrawal can be tried. The patient discontinues therapy and the family or institutional staff is asked to observe for an acceleration of decline. Generally, the rapid decline associated with AChEI withdrawal is identifiable within 1 to 2 weeks. It is important to re-

Figure 3: Effects of discontinuation and resumption of AChEI treatment. During 3 weeks on placebo (shaded area), patients previously receiving 5 mg and 10 mg daily show rapid decline in cognitive test scores. On resumption of therapy in the open-label phase, mean improvements in cognition are seen for both the group previously on placebo and those previously on active treatment. However, the discontinuation of only 3 weeks' duration appears to have completely negated all prior benefit of the 5-mg dose, since patients treated with placebo and those treated with 5 mg daily during the double-blind phase perform identically during the open-label phase.[2]

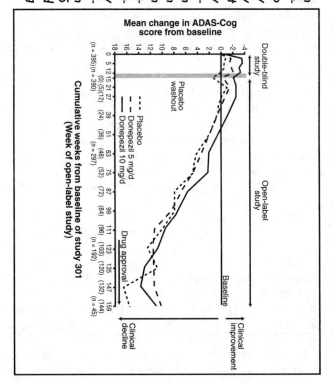

Mean change in ADAS-Cog score from baseline

Double-blind study ← → Open-label study ← → Clinical improvement

Baseline

Placebo washout

.... Placebo
– – – Donepezil 5 mg/d
—— Donepezil 10 mg/d

Drug approval

Clinical decline

Cumulative weeks from baseline of study 301 (Week of open-label study)

0   5   12 15 21 27 39 51 63 75 87 99 111 123 135 147 159
(0) (5) (12) (24) (36) (48) (52) (72) (84) (96) (103) (120) (132) (144)
(n = 395)(n = 390)   (n = 297)   (n = 192)   (n = 45)

sume therapy as early as possible when rapid functional decline is observed after withdrawal because discontinuation of donepezil for as briefly as 3 weeks is associated with irreversible losses in cognition[2] (Figure 3). Little information is available about the cognitive effects of galantamine or rivastigmine withdrawal. However, current package labeling suggests that when these agents are discontinued for more than one week, the drug should be restarted at the lowest available dosage and re-titrated to avoid severe adverse events such as esophageal rupture.

Although FDA-approved labeling states that AChEIs are indicated for mild to moderate dementia severity, some patients will continue to show benefits even in the severe stages of the illness. One clinically useful endpoint is when the patient is no longer able to contribute meaningfully to basic activities such as dressing, feeding, grooming, toileting, or bathing. For these patients, the same pattern of carefully observing function after discontinuation of therapy is warranted. Some patients will show further rapid declines in function, or worsening of behavior, which would be an indication to resume therapy.

Available Agents
Donepezil
Donepezil (Aricept®) is the most commonly prescribed drug for AD in the United States, where it was approved for marketing in late 1996. It is a piperidine-derived AChEI with high specificity for AChE. It is labeled for the treatment of mild and moderate AD.

Cognition. In a 6-month, placebo-controlled trial of donepezil,[4] approximately 16% of patients taking 5 mg daily showed at least 7 points of improvement on the 70-point Alzheimer's Disease Assessment Scale's cognitive battery (ADAS-cog). At the 10-mg daily dose, slightly more than 25% demonstrated similar improvement. Both 5-mg and 10-mg treatment groups had ADAS-cog scores superior to placebo throughout the 6-month trial. Moreover, more than 80% of treated patients showed either improvement or no decline over the 6-month trial.[4] The longest placebo-controlled AChEI experience reported to date has been 1 year.[7] Cognitive scores among donepezil-treated patients in that multicenter international trial were most improved at the 3-month point in therapy. After 1 year, cognitive test scores showed no statistically significant decline.

Donepezil has also been tested in more severely affected populations. It was associated with improved cognition relative to placebo in a 6-month trial in patients defined to have moderate-to-severe AD.[18] Treatment efficacy has been demonstrated in a clinical trial in institutionalized AD patients, with significant drug-placebo differences favoring donepezil in the measures of cognition (MMSE) and overall dementia severity (CDR-SB).[17]

Behavior. Among moderate-to-severe AD patients who did not already require psychotropic medications, donepezil was associated with improvements in behavior on the Neuropsychiatric Inventory (NPI).[18] Significant donepezil-placebo differences were identified for anxiety, apathy, and depression/dysphoria. This effect was not observed in patients already using psychotropics. In a retrospective study, patients taking donepezil were less likely to receive prescriptions for antidepressants, antipsychotics, and sedatives.[19]

Function. In comparison to a steady decline in global function among placebo-treated AD patients, donepezil-treated patients retained baseline levels of function throughout a 6-month trial.[4] In a 1-year, placebo-controlled trial, AD patients treated with donepezil had a significantly higher likelihood of maintaining ADL scores compared to placebo patients from 12 weeks onward.[20]

Dosing. Donepezil is available in 5-mg and 10-mg unscored tablets. The usual starting dose is 5 mg daily. If the agent is well tolerated with no symptomatic side effects, the dose can be increased to 10 mg daily after 4 to 6 weeks. In clinical trials, rapid increases from 5 mg to 10 mg daily were associated with a higher rate of adverse effects than the same increase after 4 weeks. Since the tablets are not scored and the half-life is long, 5 mg q.o.d. can be tried for 2 weeks if a patient experiences adverse effects on the initial dose. The rate of side effects is sufficiently low, however, that few patients need to use alternate day dosing from the outset. Similarly, alternating doses of 5 mg and 10 mg daily may be useful if a patient shows improvement but experiences intolerable side effects on the initiation of 10 mg daily dosing. Using 5 mg b.i.d. for 1 to 2 weeks can ease adverse effects associated with the transition from 5 mg to 10 mg daily. Although mean efficacy of the 5-mg and 10-mg doses was equivalent in short trials, the higher frequency of cognitive improvement on 10 mg (27% vs 16%)[4] warrants the dose increase.

Rivastigmine

Rivastigmine (Exelon®) is a carbamate-derived AChEI that was approved in the United States in 2000. Rivastigmine's activity has been reported to be highly selective for the hippocampus and cortex. In addition, rivastigmine has a relatively greater inhibitory effect on butyrylcholinesterase than on AChE, although the clinical significance of this is not clear.[21]

Cognition. In two separate 6-month, double-blind, placebo-controlled trials of rivastigmine vs placebo, cognition deteriorated in placebo-treated patients, while those treated with 6 mg to 12 mg of rivastigmine daily maintained or slightly improved from their baseline level of performance on the ADAS-cog.[5,6] Patients treated with doses of 1 mg to 4 mg daily progressed somewhat less than those on placebo, but doses less than 6 mg/day did not provide statistically significant benefit. In 6-month, placebo-controlled trials,12% to 16% of patients taking 6 mg to 12 mg of rivastigmine daily showed at least 7 points of improvement on the ADAS-cog. Treated groups had ADAS-cog scores superior to placebo throughout the 6-month trials. Approximately 55% of treated patients showed either improvement or no decline over 6 months of treatment.[5] Placebo-controlled studies of rivastigmine lasting longer than 6 months, or studies assessing treatment in more severely affected populations, have not been published. Similarly, no placebo-controlled trials of rivastigmine's impact on behavioral instruments have been published.

Function. Rivastigmine studies have used the Progressive Deterioration Scale (PDS) to assess activities of daily living. In two 6-month, double-blind studies, the PDS was relatively stable in patients treated with 6 mg to 12 mg/day of rivastigmine. This was significantly better than for 1 mg to 4 mg/day and placebo groups.[5,6]

Dosing. Rivastigmine is available in 1.5-mg, 3-mg, 4.5-mg, and 6-mg capsules, as well as in a 2 mg/mL oral solution. Patients should be started on one 1.5 mg capsule b.i.d. The dose can be raised every 4 weeks until the 6 mg b.i.d. or maximum tolerated dose is achieved. The package insert recommends that doses be given with the morning and evening meals. If significant symptoms of intolerance occur, such as vomiting or diarrhea, skipping several doses and resuming at the last tolerated dosage is advisable. Doses less than 3.0 mg b.i.d. have not demonstrated efficacy in clinical trials, so all patients should be increased to at least that dose. Intolerance of doses less than 6 mg/day is an indication to try a different member of the drug class. Although it is less convenient for both the prescribing clinician and the patient, doses need not be increased by 1.5 mg b.i.d. at each adjustment. Intermediate dosing is possible, such as using 3 mg in the morning and 4.5 mg in the evening.

Galantamine

Galantamine (Reminyl®) was approved for US distribution in 2001. The labeled mechanism of action for galantamine in the US is acetylcholinesterase inhibition, but additional evidence suggests a further direct facilitative effect on nicotinic ACh receptors. The reported effect of the nicotinic receptor modulation is to increase synaptic acetylcholine and increase release of other neurotransmitters, such as glutamate.[22] Galantamine has an approximately 10-fold selectivity for AChE compared with butyrylcholinesterase.

Cognition. In double-blind, placebo-controlled trials, galantamine doses of 8 mg b.i.d. and 12 mg b.i.d. resulted in significant improvements on the ADAS-cog in comparison with placebo. Doses of 4 mg b.i.d. did not demonstrate statistically significant differences from placebo. In a 6-month, placebo-controlled trial, approximately 16% of patients taking 24 mg of galantamine daily showed at least 7 points of improvement on the ADAS-cog. Treated groups had ADAS-cog scores superior to placebo throughout the 6-month trial. Approximately 65% of treated patients showed either improvement or no decline over 6 months of treatment.[3]

Behavior. In a 5-month, double-blind trial, 8 mg b.i.d. dosing of galantamine was associated with stable scores on the NPI. Placebo-treated patients showed statistically significant worsening over the same interval.[23]

Function. Galantamine has demonstrated beneficial effects relative to placebo on the Alzheimer's Disease Cooperative Study-ADL scale over 5 months at both 16 mg and 24 mg daily.[23] After 6 months of open-label treatment following a 6-month double-blind study, patients treated with 24 mg of galantamine daily had not declined.[3] Natural history studies and historical placebo groups suggest that significant decline on this instrument is likely over 1 year of AD without treatment.

Dosing. Galantamine is available in 4-mg, 8-mg, and 12-mg tablets, as well as in a 4 mg/mL oral solution. Patients should be started at 4 mg b.i.d., and the dose should be increased to 8 mg b.i.d. after 4 weeks. A subsequent increase to 12 mg b.i.d. may be considered if the patient tolerates the medication well after 4 more weeks. Patients with significant hepatic or renal impairments should not be increased to the 24 mg/day level. The package insert recommends dosing with morning and evening meals.[14]

Direct Comparison and Switching Studies

By early 2003, only one report had been published that directly compared the efficacy and tolerability of rivastigmine and donepezil. Mild-to-moderately impaired AD patients were randomized to donepezil or to rivastigmine in a 12-week, open-label study. At each evaluation during the study, the two treatment groups were indistinguishable in their performance on the ADAS-cog. Because 22% of the rivastigmine group discontinued therapy because of adverse effects vs 11% of the donepezil group, the investigators concluded that donepezil was the better tolerated of two equipotent agents, at least when following dosing titration schedules from the package insert.[24] Other comparative trials between donepezil and galantamine have been conducted. Although the results had not been published as this edition was going to press, preliminary reports suggest very similar overall efficacy.

There has been controversy over the value of switching from one AChEI to another. Several theoretical justifications and open-label studies have been reported.[25,26] One shortcoming of these studies is the undirectional nature of the drug changes, from donepezil to rivastigmine. Discontinuation of donepezil and improvement after institution of rivastigmine should not be interpreted as evidence of superior rivastigmine efficacy because the parallel changeovers in the opposite direction (ie, rivastigmine to donepezil) have not been studied. Further caution is warranted in interpreting these studies because of evidence that resuming treatment with the same agent after a temporary discontinuation is also associated with improvement in cognitive test scores[2] (Figure 3).

Conclusions

All three cholinesterase inhibitor drugs now in use offer similar efficacy in treating mild-to-moderate Alzheimer's disease. For all three agents, a minority of patients will show easily discernible cognitive improvements, but stabilization of the course for 6 to 12 months is the most common outcome of therapy. Behavioral and functional symptoms may also show benefit. Differences in mechanism of action have not translated into clinically meaningful differences in efficacy between these agents. There is converging evidence that persistent treatment with members of this class can result in reduced risk for institutionalization. In general use, AChEIs are safe and well tolerated. Gastrointestinal side effects are most common, but are ameliorated by slow dose titration. Intolerance of one medication in the class does not predict intolerance to others, but there is insufficient information in the literature to support routine switching between agents to achieve greater efficacy.

References

1. Doody RS, Stevens JC, Beck C, et al: Practice parameter: Management of dementia (an evidence-based review): report of the Quality Standards Subcommittee of the American Academy of Neurology. *Neurology* 2001;56:1154-1166.

2. Doody RS, Geldmacher DS, Gordon B, et al, for the Donepezil Study Group: Open-label, multicenter, phase 3 extension study of the safety and efficacy of donepezil in patients with Alzheimer disease. *Arch Neurol* 2001;58:427-433.

3. Raskind MA, Peskind ER, Wessel T, et al: Galantamine in AD: a 6-month, randomized, placebo- controlled trial with a six-month extension. *Neurology* 2000;54:2261-2268.

4. Rogers SL, Farlow MR, Doody RS, et al: A 24-week double-blind, placebo-controlled trial of donepezil in patients with Alzheimer's disease. *Neurology* 1998a;50:136-145.

5. Corey-Bloom J, Anand R, Veach J, for the ENA 713 B352 Study Group: A randomized trial evaluating the efficacy and safety of ENA 713 (rivastigmine tartrate), a new acetylcholinesterase inhibitor, in patients with mild to moderately severe Alzheimer's disease. *Int J Geriatr Psychopharmacol* 1998;1:55-65.

6. Rösler M, Anand R, Cicin-Sain A, et al: Efficacy and safety of rivastigmine in patients with Alzheimer's disease: international randomised controlled trial. *BMJ* 1999;318:633-638.

7. Winblad B, Engedal K, Soininen H, et al: A 1-year, randomized, placebo-controlled study of donepezil in patients with mild to moderate AD. *Neurology* 2001;57:489-495.

8. Jann MW, Shirley KL, Small GW: Clinical pharmacokinetics and pharmacodynamics of cholinesterase inhibitors. *Clin Pharmacokinet* 2002;41:719-739.

9. Knopman DS, Schneider L, Davis K: Long-term tacrine (Cognex) treatment: effects on nursing home placement and mortality, Tacrine Study Group. *Neurology* 1996;47(1):166-77.

10. Lopez OL, Becker JT, Wisniewski S, et al: Cholinesterase inhibitor treatment alters the natural history of Alzheimer's disease. *J Neurol Neurosurg Psychiatry* 2002;72:310-314.

11. Geldmacher DS, Provenzano G, McRae T, et al: Donepezil is associated with delayed nursing home placement in patients with Alzheimer's disease. *J Am Geriatr Soc* (in press).

12. Karlawish JH, Klocinski JL, Merz J, et al: Caregivers' preferences for the treatment of patients with Alzheimer's disease. *Neurology* 2000;55:1008-10014.

13. Grutzendler J, Morris JC: Cholinesterase inhibitors for Alzheimer's disease. *Drugs* 2001;61:41-50.

14. Reminyl [Package insert]. Titusville, NJ, Janssen Pharmaceutica, 2001.

15. Exelon [Package insert]. East Hanover, NJ, Novartis, 2001.

16. Aricept [Package insert]. Teaneck, NJ, Eisai Inc, 2001.

17. Tariot PN, Cummings JL, Katz JR, et al: A randomized, double-blind, placebo-controlled study of the efficacy and safety of donepezil patients with Alzheimer's disease in the nursing home setting. *J Am Geriatr Soc* 2001;49:1590-1599.

18. Feldman H, Gauthier S, Hecker J, et al: A 24-week, randomized, double-blind study of donepezil in moderate to severe Alzheimer's disease. *Neurology* 57:613-620.

19. Small G, Donohue J, Brooks R: An economic evaluation of donepezil in the treatment of Alzheimer's disease. *Clin Ther* 1998; 20:838-850.

20. Mohs RC, Doody RS, Morris JC, et al: A 1-year, placebo-controlled preservation of function survival study of donepezil in AD patients. *Neurology* 2001;57:481-488.

21. Weinstock M: Selectivity of cholinesterase inhibition. Clinical implications for the treatment of Alzheimer's disease *CNS Drugs* 1999;12:307-323.

22. Maelicke A, Samochocki M, Jostock R, et al: Allosteric sensitization of nicotinic receptors by galantamine, a new treatment strategy for Alzheimer's disease. *Biol Psychiatry* 2001;49:279-288.

23. Tariot PN, Solomon PR, Morris JC, et al: A 5-month, randomized, placebo-controlled trial of galantamine in AD. *Neurology* 2000;54:2269-2276.

24. Wilkinson DG, Passmore AP, Bullock R, et al: A multinational, randomised, 12-week comparative study of donepezil and rivastigmine in patients with mild to moderate Alzheimer's disease. *Int J Clin Pract* 2002;56:441-446.

25. Auriacombe S, Pere J-J, Loria-Kanza Y, et al: Efficacy and safety of patients with Alzheimer's disease who failed to benefit from treatment with donepezil. *Curr Med Research Opin* 2002;18:129-138.

26. Bullock R, Connolly C: Switching cholinesterase inhibitor therapy in Alzheimer's disease—donepezil to rivastigmine, is it worth it? *Int J Geriatr Psychiatry* 2002;17:288-289.

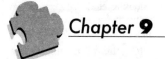

Chapter 9

Treatment of Behavioral Symptoms

Alzheimer's disease (AD) is usually defined by progressive memory loss. In addition to cognitive changes, most AD patients also develop noncognitive behavioral symptoms during the illness. These symptoms are reviewed in Chapter 3. This chapter reviews the general principles of treating behavioral symptoms in AD, as well as pharmacologic and non-pharmacologic approaches to common adverse behaviors. Behavioral symptoms are extremely stressful to caregivers, often much more so than cognitive decline. In addition, noncognitive features of the disease are common triggers for urgent calls to the doctor's office and long-term care decisions.

Evaluation of Acute Behavior Changes

Behavioral symptoms usually emerge gradually and evolve slowly over the course of dementia. For acute, severe, or first-ever episodes of adverse behaviors, an urgent or emergency evaluation is warranted. Agitation, acute psychosis, and aggressive behaviors are commonly associated with delirium caused by occult general medical conditions (Chapter 4). Since delirium usually reflects a life-threatening underlying medical illness, evaluation for its sources takes priority. Dehydration, urinary tract infection, urinary retention, pain, sleep deprivation, hunger, constipation, and infectious or inflammatory processes are all possibilities. The evaluation should, therefore, include a careful physical examination and general metabolic work-up for sources of acute delirium. Laboratory assessment should include complete blood count, full blood chemistry profile (eg, SMA-20), urinalysis, chest x-ray, and arterial blood gases (ABG). Oximetry for oxygen saturation is not an ideal alternative to ABG, because it does not assess blood pH, but it can be done while awaiting other results to determine how much supplemental oxygen is needed. More detailed discussions of evaluation and management of delirium in older adults are available in the literature.[1,2]

In addition to the medical assessment, physicians must consider the family's ability to maintain the patient safely at home. Similarly, the risk for caregiver injury should be a factor in the acute treatment and disposition plans. Admitting the patient, even involuntarily, to a locked psychiatric ward is sometimes the only safe alternative for patients and caregivers.

Drug Treatment in the Older Demented Population

Changes in physiology associated with aging make drug treatment more challenging in older adults.[3] Since AD and other dementias are so strongly associated with old age, it is worth reviewing some of these issues. Although drug absorption is generally not affected by aging, drug distribution is altered through several mechanisms. The most important are reductions in lean body mass and total body water, with a concomitant increase in total body fat. This is especially important for central nervous system-(CNS) acting drugs, which tend to be lipophilic to pass through the blood-brain barrier. Two direct effects of these lipophilic properties are a delay in reaching steady state and an extended half-life in older adults compared with younger ones. For example, the half-life of diazepam (Valium®), a benzodiazepine anxiolytic frequently prescribed for agitation in dementia patients, is extended approximately 4-fold in older adults.[4] As a result, the cumulative effect of repeated diazepam doses in an elderly patient is failure to achieve the desired effects quickly, followed by delayed sedation and confusion. These complications may emerge gradually over 1 or more weeks. The adverse effect then clears very slowly because of the slow pace of elimination of the drug accumulated in fatty tissues, as well as the protracted effect of its active metabolites. For more water-soluble and protein-bound agents, the volume of distribution may actually be reduced and half-life shortened, resulting in a reduced ability to achieve steady state with conventional dose intervals. The route of elimination also influences drug therapy in older adults. Generally, renal elimination is progressively reduced with age, even with stable serum creatinine levels,[3] but hepatic metabolism is much more variable. Nonetheless, hepatic clearance can be significantly altered by concomitant medications, including alcohol and over-the-counter agents, which induce or inhibit metabolic pathways within the liver. Idiosyncratic responses of the aged brain can further complicate these factors. For example, many older adults respond with paradoxical agitation to sedative-hypnotic agents.[3] Benzodiazepines have also been associated with falls and impaired psychomotor performance in older adults.[5,6]

In addition to the effects of age, brain disease may unpredictably alter drug response. Significant neuronal loss exists in AD among the nuclei that supply acetylcholine (ACh), norepinephrine (NE), serotonin (5-HT), and dopamine (DA) to the cerebral cortex. Variably reported losses also exist in intrinsic cortical transmitters like gamma-aminobutyric acid (GABA). These losses are probably the basis for many behavioral symptoms in AD. Neuropsychopharmacologic agents are designed to alter neurotransmitter balance in the synapse, usually by acting on one of these transmitter systems. However, pharmacologic manipulation of that transmitter can have far-reaching and unpredictable effects on behavior. Normal brain function depends on carefully balanced interactions between excitatory and inhibitory neurotransmitter effects at presynaptic and postsynaptic locations, all mediated through several receptor types and signal transduction cascades. With a disease-related imbalance in transmitter activity, and presumably a physiologic attempt to compensate, the responses to medications become more unpredictable. This intrinsic variability requires that the prescriber pay careful and regular attention to the effectiveness of treatment, as well as to adverse events, in both acute and chronic time scales.

Principles of Rational Neuropsychopharmacology

Physicians generally treat behavioral symptoms in AD with the same medications they use when these symptoms appear in other neurologic or psychiatric diseases. Therefore, the approach outlined in this chapter can also be useful for other dementia states, as well as for behavioral syndromes following stroke or traumatic brain injury. These principles are depicted in Table 1.

Identify

The first step in this approach to psychopharmacology is to clearly identify the target symptoms. For example, the common complaint of agitation in AD follows several distinct behavioral patterns (Chapter 3). Furthermore, agitation can arise from multiple and sometimes simultaneous causes. To select the best therapy for a particular patient, it is therefore inappropriate to consider all agitation in the same way. In contrast, it is useful to translate the complaint of agitation into specific behaviors, such as physical aggression or pacing. Similarly, specific treatment goals for depression can be operationally defined. Examples include targeting increased total sleep hours for complaints of

Table 1: Principles of Rational Neuropsychopharmacology

- Identify the problem
- Specify the target behavior
- Quantify the symptoms
- Subtract precipitating factors
- Select the appropriate agent
- Use sequential monotherapy
- Monitor results and adjust treatment accordingly
- Make 1 adjustment at a time

poor sleep initiation, or reducing the frequency of crying as an indicator of successfully treating low mood. Generally, targeting one problem behavior at a time is a more fruitful approach than trying to normalize a wide range of problems at once.

Quantify

Quantify the target behavior once it is identified. For routine clinical use, grading the frequency of the problem behavior, its severity, or both, is usually adequate. Caregivers (both family and institutional) should keep a diary of the problem behavior that has been identified as the treatment target. Without consistent monitoring of specific behaviors, reductions in adverse behaviors can be overlooked and treatment efficacy undervalued. This is especially true when residual behavioral problems persist after treatment. For example, the prescriber may decide the selected treatment was ineffective if he or she receives word that the patient is 'still agitated,' when, in fact, 4 moderate physical assaults per week are reduced to 1 or 2 episodes of mild verbal aggression per week.

Subtract

Many difficult behaviors are triggered by external factors, such as interpersonal conflicts, environmental stress, pain, or adverse effects of other drugs. Identifying these triggers and 'subtracting' them from the patient's experience are essential steps in reducing problem behaviors.

Diurnal patterns or other systematic variations in symptoms are clues to external causes of problem behaviors and should be tracked carefully. When these triggers are identified, physicians should take steps to reduce or eliminate them. Nighttime agitation frequently stems from mild sensory deprivation, complicated by a day of relative physical and mental inactivity. Better lighting[7] and referral to a day program[8] may be more successful than drugs for this problem. Another example is large family gatherings, which may overwhelm the demented person, leading to anxiety, frustration, and tearfulness. Recognizing these patterns allows the family to alter its style of interaction and focus on smaller, quieter get-togethers. Medication use should also be reviewed as a contributor to altered behavior. For instance, over-the-counter sleep aids or cough-and-cold preparations with anticholinergic properties can lead to paradoxical agitation in AD patients.

Select an Agent

Choosing the medication most likely to help the patient is the reason for going through the steps above. Many prescribers simply respond to agitation with the same treatment in most patients. Recent trials suggest that this approach has no better than a random chance of succeeding. Carefully evaluating the roots of a behavioral problem can increase the medication success rate. For instance, agitation from boredom and disengagement may respond less well to antipsychotic drugs than to antidepressants. In contrast, agitated behaviors from paranoid delusions or low-grade hallucinations are a strong indication for antipsychotics.

The side-effect profile warrants thought in drug selection. For example, fluoxetine (Prozac®) is a potent antidepressant, but it can have alerting or activating properties. Those properties can make it a poor choice for people who have agitation symptoms as part of their depression and dementia, but it can be a good choice for the inactive, amotivated patient with depressive features. Sometimes side effects can be used to the patient's advantage. Olanzapine (Zyprexa®) is an antipsychotic agent with potent sedating side effects. For the AD patient with nighttime hallucinations and poor sleep onset, olanzapine can treat both symptoms, avoiding the need for a second agent. Caution is still warranted, however, since anticholinergically mediated confusion may offset the benefit, especially if the patient does not fall asleep. Although antipsychotic drugs usually help relieve adverse behaviors, they can also provoke extrapyramidal signs or apathetic changes that limit the person's ability to behave well, leading to a net negative effect. This approach to treating problem behaviors increases the likelihood of success and minimizes the risk to the patient for unnecessary side effects or delayed access to the most adequate treatment.

Sequential Monotherapy

The central concept of sequential monotherapy is that one agent is used for a targeted behavior until: (1) efficacy is reached, (2) the side effects are intolerable, or (3) the maximum recommended or labeled dose is achieved. A common error in dementia neuropsychopharmacology is to use too many agents, at doses too low, for too short an interval. When the clinician simultaneously initiates more than 1 new agent and side effects emerge or the behavior paradoxically worsens, it is difficult to determine which drug is the culprit. Also, because of the complex modulatory influences on synapses, neurotransmitter-based treatments may be slow to develop efficacy. The 6-

to 8-week lag in efficacy for antidepressants is a well-recognized example of giving the agent time to work. Furthermore, many prescribers set an internal or arbitrary threshold for their maximum prescribed dose of a particular agent, especially in older patients. In doing so, they may restrict the efficacy of an otherwise useful medication. This deprives the patient of the opportunity to benefit from an appropriate drug solely because of an inadequate dose. The most physiologically justified threshold to determine that a dose is too high is the development of persistent, intolerable side effects. These side effects may be something that the patient notices, like nausea, or something that the clinician notices, like extrapyramidal signs.

Physicians must recognize that the principles of sequential monotherapy support the basic tenets of geriatric pharmacology, which are to use low doses and gradual dose increments. This is often phrased as *start low, go slow*. The use of a single agent is ideal from the standpoint of geriatrics because it limits the risk for systemic drug interactions, as well as the more subtle problems associated with competing neurotransmitter effects in the brain. This approach does, however, require the prescriber to thoroughly understand the CNS mechanism of action, as well as the systemic side-effect profile of each drug chosen for the patient.

There are clearly times when just one drug is inadequate to meet the patient's needs. One example might be crippling anxiety related to fearfulness about an unfamiliar environment. While buspirone (BuSpar®), trazodone, or selective serotonin reuptake inhibitor (SSRI) antidepressants may be useful for long-term relief, they are too slow to reduce distress immediately. In this situation, acute use of low-dose, short half-life benzodiazepines (eg, lorazepam) is initially indicated to supplement more chronic suppressive therapy. Monitor the patient carefully to limit potential adverse effects of benzodiazepine accumulation, and reduce the dosage as the symptoms abate.

Monitor and Adjust

Regardless of which agent is chosen, the prescriber must monitor the therapy for both effectiveness and toxicity. The interval for reassessment and dose adjustment depends on many factors, but the choice should reflect the expected time of response to the drug. It is not the target symptom that determines how long it takes the medicine to work. Therefore, the severity of the problem, and not the type of symptom, should dictate the aggressiveness of the medication plan. An acutely acting agent for anxiety, such as a benzodiazepine, can be expected to have its effect within the first or second dose. If the patient fails to respond within that time, the physician must reassess either the agent or the dose. In contrast, buspirone may take several weeks to target the same symptom complex. Table 2 lists consensus opinions on how long different classes of medicines take to show meaningful results.[9] Caregivers should be encouraged to keep notes on the target behavior. Dissatisfaction despite improvement in the target symptom may mean that a different symptom is causing the distress. In contrast, it is possible to overshoot the target symptom. A sedative used to promote sleep onset can result in daytime somnolence if overdosed.

Prescribers should frequently reassess whether the problem behavior still needs drug treatment. Difficult behaviors in AD present a moving target. They change not only with disease progression, but also with increasing caregiver sophistication and reliance on community services. Furthermore, initial control of a problem behavior often requires higher doses than maintenance suppression. For example, after successful crisis management, a clinician can reduce the dose or discontinue medications. One of the most common errors in prescribing for behavioral symptoms is continuing therapy long after the primary indication passes. Because of this, regulations governing psychotropic drug use in long-term care

Table 2: Defining Adequate Treatment Trials of Medications[9]

How long to try a first medication before increasing dose, switching drugs, or adding another drug if the response to treatment is inadequate

Medication	Shortest interval	Longest interval
Antipsychotic	4-7 days	2-4 weeks
Benzodiazepine	3-4 days	1-3 weeks
Buspirone	1.5-2.5 weeks	4-6 weeks
Divalproex	1-2 weeks	3-6 weeks
SSRI*	10-14 days	4-6 weeks
Trazodone*	10-14 days	3-4 weeks

*Also see Table 3 for dose titration recommendations.

mandate a regular reappraisal of the indications and dosages of agents prescribed for behavioral problems.

Drug doses for behavioral symptoms should generally be lowered incrementally, rather than stopped abruptly, except in cases of serious side effects. Tapering lets prescribers determine the minimum effective dose even when discontinuation is interrupted by the reemergence of symptoms. If the target behavior reappears, the dose should be raised, not to the original dose, but to the last effective dose.

Given the complexity of behavioral disturbances associated with dementia, many patients take multiple psychotropic medicines. When prescribers want to change regimens because of incomplete efficacy, they should adjust only one agent at a time. That way, both successes and emergent adverse events can be tracked. It also allows the prescriber to be more informed for the next adjustment. A common problem is making 2 dosage changes simultaneously. If the patient is more agitated in 2 days, the cause could be either drug, their interaction at the new doses, or a completely unrelated event. The prescriber, unfortunately, has no way of knowing the exact cause and then must reduce the dosages of both agents to the starting points. The patient, caregiver, and prescriber then lose time looking for a more successful treatment approach.

Nonpharmacologic Approaches

As noted above, many problem behaviors have environmental antecedents. No medication regimen is completely effective if precipitating factors are not addressed. The expertise for teaching or applying these interventions frequently lies with nonphysician health providers, other professionals, and community agencies. The American Academy of Neurology practice parameter for management of dementia emphasizes the importance of training and dementia-specific education for individuals who provide care for patients with dementing illnesses.[10] Chapter 10 addresses the roles of these providers and appropriate referral patterns. Some basic approaches should be familiar to every clinician who works with demented patients and their families.

Communication Strategies

Alzheimer's disease is associated with a loss of language ability, which is subtle but present even in early stages. The cognitive deficits of AD also limit the speed and capacity of processing information. Caregivers must recognize that these changes combine to interfere with the patients' ability to understand a complex environment. In addition, many AD patients have age-related deficits in hearing and vision that compromise the sensory inputs to cognition. Therefore, hearing and vision should be tested and optimized in patients with possible dementia.

Compensatory strategies are necessary to enhance communication and to reduce patient frustrations associated with poor environmental comprehension. Specific curricula have been developed to assist caregivers in developing these skills.[11] Facial expression is important for conveying meaning in conversation. Face-to-face conversation with good eye contact often facilitates understanding. This requires a change in style for many families, who have developed conversational habits such as speaking 'over-the-shoulder' or across a room while both conversation partners look at the television, rather than at each other. Attention problems may limit the AD patient's ability to cope with multiple stimuli. Therefore, important conversations should be conducted in the least distracting environment possible. This often means turning off the television or moving to a quieter room in a busy household. The same deficit creates difficulty for the patient in coping with multiple conversations, such as at social gatherings. The typical patient response is to become withdrawn and silent when the information exceeds his or her capacity for processing. However, some individuals become agitated and belligerent.

In speaking with the AD patient, family members should keep sentences direct and brief. Complex sentence structures reduce comprehension. Open-ended questions, such as, "What would you like for dinner?", are more difficult than single-choice questions, such as, "Would you like chicken tonight?" Many family members may increase agitation and irritability through well-intentioned but counterproductive actions. One example is a quiz approach to memory failures. This occurs when the patient fails to recall an event and the caregiver offers a series of questions to 'help' the affected person remember, such as, "Don't you remember what we did last Sunday?" Instead of facilitating memory, these questions often frustrate the patient. Caregivers should avoid confronting patients with their memory failures. When a patient does not understand, a common caregiver response is to speak louder, as if hearing rather than comprehension is the problem. Patients may interpret the louder, more intense voice as being 'yelled at,' and respond with anger in turn. Caregivers must simplify the content, rather than raise the volume, when the patient does not understand.

Sleep and Activity

Sleep difficulties are common in AD and often start a cascade of worsening behavior symptoms and increasing caregiver stress.[12] Several factors influence sleep in demented persons. Generally, both the total hours of sleep and sleep efficiency decrease with aging.[13] Cognitively intact people alter behaviors to match the changing sleep patterns by varying bedtimes or taking naps. In dementia, however, the caregiver, rather than the patient, dictates sleep patterns, sometimes leading to a mismatch between the patient's activities and sleep needs. Because of apathy and diminished ability to initiate behaviors, many people with AD sit passively, often in front of a television, throughout the day. Their cognitive impairments make it difficult to process the high-content stream of information from the television, so they withdraw from it and doze intermittently through the day. Caregivers value this because they can accomplish their chores without interference. By the time the caregiver is tired from managing the household during the day, the patient is well rested and energetic. This leads to conflict and poor nighttime sleep for both parties, and triggers an erosion of the day-night cycle. Caregivers often seek sedative-hypnotic drugs for the patient. *It is important to recognize and communicate that hypnotics generally act only to promote sleep onset, not prolong sleep duration.* Hypnotic drugs often simply push the patient's period of wakefulness even deeper into the night, magnifying the problems of the next day for both patient and caregiver.

When this cycle of sleep disturbance emerges, families should find more suitable daytime activities for patients. An appropriate set of activities is one that engages the affected person mentally or emotionally and promotes daytime wakefulness. Passive activities, such as watching television or listening to the radio, are usually not adequate if the person cannot stay awake. Physical activities, such as walks or shopping trips, are ideal because they consume energy and stimulate the senses. Humans are social creatures and most respond well to comfortable social interactions. Social encounters, like lunch with the affected person's friends, can temporarily relieve the caregiver from the stress of providing care while affording a positive outlet for the patient. In addition to increased daytime activity, other useful nonpharmacologic strategies include setting regular sleep and waking times, limiting daytime sleeping, avoiding fluid intake in the evening, and using calming bedtime rituals.[14] Restricting daytime caffeine intake may also help.[9] Generally, clinical experience suggests that implementation of these behavioral approaches is more successful than drug treatments, particularly over-the-counter agents for sleep. More detailed descriptions of drug approaches to sleep disturbance appear below.

Nutrition

Weight loss almost always accompanies dementia.[15] This may reflect neurogenic loss of appetite, loss of flavor sensation, apathy, depression, and many other factors. Patients who prepare their own meals may simply forget to do so, or forget how. Mealtime can also become a source of family conflict that further diminishes feeding. The AD patient, inactive during the day, is probably less hungry and has reduced caloric demands in comparison with lifetime habits. When the well-meaning caregiver urges the patient to eat, it can lead to frustration and conflicts. When the patient loses weight, the caregiver often provides larger servings. Placing more food on the plate does not generally increase the amount that the person eats; it only increases the amount of food left behind, further frustrating the caregiver.

Several interventions can ameliorate this pattern. Meals should be kept low-key and free of conflict. Small, frequent servings can also help increase intake. Foods should be focused on patient favorites, rather than the strict heart-healthy diets promoted in many older adults. Apraxia interferes with utensil use, so food choices should be amenable to using fingers and the caregiver should allow the patient to dispense with silverware when necessary. A dietitian may be helpful as a part of an interdisciplinary plan to help the family optimize the patient's nutritional status (Chapter 10).[16]

Day Care

Adult day programs offer many families a simple and cost-effective solution to the preceding problems. Day-care programs provide a safe and stimulating environment designed for the needs of cognitively impaired individuals. Well-run programs focus on activities that are fulfilling to their clients, keeping them active, engaged, and awake during the day. Most also provide well-balanced nutrition. Perhaps more importantly, they allow the caregiver a respite from the rigors of providing around-the-clock care. There are very few controlled studies on the effect of day-care programs for dementia, but families often report they are an important part of coping with the stress of caregiving. Day care does not appear to have significant effects on cognition, activities of daily living, or overall behavioral disturbances, but it does provide a direct benefit to families by reducing caregiver exhaustion and delaying nursing home placement for many patients.[8] Local outlets of the Office on Aging or Alzheimer's Association frequently maintain up-to-date lists of day programs available in the community.

Driving

Dementia-related driving impairment is not really a behavioral problem, but is addressed here because it requires nonpharmacologic approaches to management by the physician and family. Restriction of motor-vehicle driving privileges is traumatic for many families and can trigger behavioral difficulties, including anger, agitation, and depression. The American Psychiatric Association's practice guideline for treatment of AD and other dementias[14] states that the physician should advise the patient and family that even mild dementia impairs driving and increases the risk for accidents. The guideline recommends that mildly impaired patients limit or discontinue driving. Furthermore, patients with a greater degree of visuospatial, dysexecutive, or apractic impairments should be restricted from driving earlier in the course of dementia. Patients with moderate or more severe impairments (eg, those who cannot prepare simple meals, perform household chores, or complete simple home repairs) should discontinue driving. The American Academy of Neurology practice parameter for driving in dementia is somewhat more restrictive, recommending that driving be discontinued when a person is classified as having mild AD, based on formal criteria such as the Clinical Dementia Rating Scale (see Chapter 3). If driving is restricted, the physician may also consider restricting similarly risky activities, such as using power tools or lawn mowers. Since family members usually enforce driving bans, they must be informed of the decision. The physician can support the family's enforcement by providing a prescription that states "Do Not Drive."[14]

It is often useful for the physician to tell the patient of his or her concerns about cognitive performance, and instruct the patient not to drive until the evaluation is complete. This softens the initial blow of the restriction, since it may be temporary, and allows an easier transition to a permanent driving ban if the illness is irreversible or progressive. When additional information about driving skill is necessary to determine a recommendation to continue or cease driving, referral to an occupational therapy/driver's evaluation program is warranted (Chapter 10). These programs may also offer driver rehabilitation for borderline cases, though it is unlikely to have any long-term use in a patient with progressive cognitive decline.

Pharmacologic Approaches

This chapter has already addressed the general principles of pharmacotherapy and basic nonpharmacologic approaches for behavioral symptoms in dementia. It will now outline specific drug approaches to common emotional and behavioral problems. Many idiosyncrasies exist in the choice of agents for behavioral symptoms. Consensus approaches will be cited wherever possible, but this is a rapidly evolving field. There have been dramatic changes, both in the clinical approach to these symptoms and agents available to treat them, in just the last 10 years. New drugs will continue to reach the market. The recommendations for agents in this section must therefore be considered in light of the possibility that other drugs, some superior and some not, have become available since publication of this edition.

Depression

As noted in Chapter 3, depressive symptoms are common in AD. They can presage the development of cognitive deficits, or occur in response to losses in ability and independence. Depressive symptoms can worsen cognition, magnify functional disability, exacerbate other behavioral difficulties (eg, agitated depression), and diminish quality of life. The threshold for diagnosing major depression need not be crossed for the effects on quality of life and function to be seen. Therefore, symptomatic approaches should be considered even if a formal diagnosis of major depression is not applied. Besides resolution of low mood, the goals of therapy for depression in dementia should include improvement in cognition and reduction of apathy.[14]

Studies of the efficacy of antidepressant agents in dementia are complicated by a number of factors, but it appears that mood can be improved in many individuals. There is little evidence that any one conventional antidepressant is better against typical depressive or vegetative symptoms. The choice of agents must then rest on side effects, ease of use, cost, and the potential for drug interactions. Selective serotonin reuptake inhibitors, which include citalopram (Celexa™), fluoxetine (Prozac®), paroxetine (Paxil®), and sertraline (Zoloft®), generally have favorable side-effect profiles when compared with other antidepressant classes. Cyclic agents, such as amitriptyline, nortriptyline, and imipramine, among others, have a higher risk for cardiovascular effects and are generally more anticholinergic, limiting their use in AD. Imipramine, for example, has been implicated in worsening cognition in AD patients.[17] Trazodone is less anticholinergic and has fewer cardiac risks than other heterocyclic agents, but can trigger priapism in men and is often potently sedating. These sedative properties can help the patient if sleep difficulties complicate the depressive picture. The restrictive drug and dietary prohibitions associated with antidepressant monoamine oxidase inhibitors (MAOIs) make them generally unsuitable for use in dementia.

Selective serotonin reuptake inhibitors are an appropriate first choice in most patients because of their side-effect advantages, but prominent interindividual variability exists in response to SSRIs. Both sertraline and citalopram offer a relatively neutral effect on arousal and favorable drug interaction profiles, making them preferable in most patients. Fluoxetine is more generally arousing, which can cause agitation in some patients, but can be favorable in others who are more apathetic or underaroused. In contrast, paroxetine is somewhat more anticholinergic and sedating in most pa-

Table 3: Dosing of SSRI Antidepressants and Trazodone[14]

Agent	Initial dose (q.d.)
Citalopram*	10-20 mg
Fluoxetine	5-10 mg
Paroxetine	5-10 mg
Sertraline	25 mg
Trazodone	25-50 mg

*Information derived from package insert, not reference 14.

tients. Any of these agents, however, can cause sedation or restlessness and an adverse response to one does not necessarily predict a similar response to other members of the class. Typical dosing options are outlined in Table 3.

Treatment should generally continue for at least 6 months after depressive target symptoms abate, and physicians should be sensitive to nondrug factors that help with successful discontinuation. These include seasonal effects (it is better to stop therapy in the spring rather than winter or fall) and losses, such as death anniversaries. To discontinue antidepressants, taper their use over weeks. If symptoms re-emerge during the taper, resume therapy at the last effective dose and continue for 6 to 12 months. If an AD patient twice fails antidepressant dose tapers, chronic therapy is probably necessary.

Anxiety

Anxiety frequently accompanies depression in demented patients. In those cases, treatment should proceed for depression. More rarely, generalized or chronic anxi-

Interval between dose increases	Maximum dose
1-2 weeks	40 mg/day
2-3 weeks	40-60 mg/day
1-2 weeks	40-60 mg/day
1-2 weeks	150-200 mg/day
5-7 days	300-400 mg/day

ety complicates AD without concurrent mood effects. This is identified by persistent facial or verbal expressions of worry, nervousness, or fear without low mood. Somatic symptoms, such as nonspecific headache or gastrointestinal symptoms, often relate to less intense anxiety. In contrast, acute anxiety is typically triggered by anticipation of events, such as visits to the doctor's office or impending travel. Environmental circumstances, like parties or visiting grandchildren, can also act as triggers.

Benzodiazepines are appropriate for acute short-term anxiety severe enough for drug intervention. Lorazepam (Ativan®), 0.5 mg to 1.0 mg, is a good starting point for intermittent or as-needed use, since it features relatively rapid absorption and quick clearance.[9] Oxazepam (Serax®), 7.5 mg to 15 mg, is less useful for as-needed dosing because it is absorbed more slowly.[14] Either of these agents, or longer-acting agents like clonazepam (Klonopin®), are used to maintain a patient's symptoms at an acceptable level while long-term management strategies are adopted. Diazepam, though a popular agent, is characterized by slow clearance, and further complicated by the prolonged effect of active metabolites. It is generally not recommended in the elderly. Few patients require, or benefit from, chronic benzodiazepine use. Because of their adverse safety profile, members of the benzodiazepine class are not recommended for long-term use.[9] If benzodiazepines are used consistently over weeks, they should be tapered, rather than discontinued abruptly, because of a high risk of withdrawal effects.

When regular or daily doses of benzodiazepines are required to maintain acceptable symptom levels, then a long-term agent is indicated. Buspirone, beginning at 5 mg b.i.d., and increasing to 50 mg to 60 mg daily in divided doses, is the recommendation of one consensus process.[9] Many clinicians prefer SSRIs or trazodone as alternatives because of their once-daily dosing. Typical antidepressant doses are appropriate. Lorazepam can still be used for intermittent anxiety exacerbations in addition to chronic anxiolytic therapy.

Psychosis

Psychosis represents a breakdown in the patient's ability to evaluate reality. By definition, psychotic thoughts are, therefore, irrational. Families will often try to dissuade the affected person from the delusion or hallucination by using rational arguments. This is doomed to failure, and often exacerbates agitation (see below). The psychotic thoughts are the actual experience of the individual, and since they are the result of impaired reality testing, they will not be altered by the caregiver's perception of reality. Therefore, if psychotic symptoms are troubling to the patient, drug therapy is required. In contrast, if the psychotic features are not a problem for the patient, support for the caregiver and simple observation are adequate. The goal of antipsychotic therapy is to reduce psychosis, with resultant decreased agitation and increased comfort for the patient and caregiver.[14]

Table 4: Dosing of Antipsychotic Agents in Elderly Demented Patients with Behavioral Disturbances Requiring Antipsychotic Drug Therapy[9,14] (doses are daily total, in mg)

Agent	Initial dose	Average target dose	Highest recommended dose
Haloperidol	0.5-1.0	1.5-2.0	2-7
Olanzapine	2.5-5.0	5.0-7.5	12.5-15
Quetiapine*	12.5-25	50-100	150-300
Risperidone	0.25-0.5	0.5-1.5	2-6

*Quetiapine usually requires twice daily or more frequent dosing. Quetiapine information is derived from clinical experience and package labeling, not references 9 or 14.

Severe acute psychosis may be associated with physical violence or other dangerous behaviors. In such cases, conventional high-potency antipsychotic agents, such as haloperidol (Haldol®), 0.5 mg or more, are indicated.[9] They can be administered parenterally in an emergency and should be used while the clinician evaluates for the acute medical causes of the behavioral exacerbation (see above).

Haloperidol, like most high-potency antipsychotics, carries a substantial risk for causing extrapyramidal motor signs (EPS) in doses required to suppress psychosis. For chronic use, atypical agents are, therefore, preferable. Risperidone (Risperdal®) is an effective agent for adverse behaviors in dementia and appears to have a lower risk for extrapyramidal complications than haloperidol. Clinical experience suggests that elderly demented patients requiring dosages in excess of 2 to 3 mg daily are likely to develop EPS. Olanzapine is often more acutely sedating, which makes it useful when psychosis is more difficult at night. Quetiapine (Seroquel®) is effective against psychotic symptoms and does not worsen cognition.[18] It is mildly sedating and has a low risk for EPS in general psychiatric populations; twice daily dosing is typical. For patients with prominent parkinsonian features, or intolerance to other atypical antipsychotic agents because of EPS, clozapine may be a useful alternative. Clozapine (Clozaril®) is more difficult to manage because of mandatory white blood cell count monitoring. It is most often used in specialty clinics where the concentration of cases makes monitoring more cost-effective. Dosing of these agents is reviewed in Table 4.

Anger and Aggression

Anger and aggression are characterized by hostile feelings, acts, or words directed at other people, typically caregivers. It can be very difficult to establish a drug treatment plan for these behaviors because they are most often triggered by interaction with other people. Personal care activities, such as bathing or feeding, are a common precipitant. Aggression can also emerge when the demented individual's desires are frustrated, such as being prevented from leaving the house when he or she wants to take a walk (or wander). Other precipitating factors include a sense of being overwhelmed by a situation or misinterpreting the environment.[9] Avoiding or restructuring the trigger event is a mandatory nonpharmacologic first step in treating these behaviors, but in many cases it is insufficient to completely eliminate the problem.

Little consensus exists on the best drug approach to aggression and violence. When acute suppression of aggressive or assaultive behaviors is needed, conventional high-potency neuroleptics (eg, haloperidol) or risperidone are indicated if oral approaches are justified; olanzapine, quetiapine, and trazodone can also be considered.[9] Depending on the severity of the problem and the risk to others, parenteral high-potency antipsychotic drugs may be necessary. Acute or short-term use of benzodiazepines can complement other approaches, but are not the primary solution. New or acute interpersonal violence always warrants an evaluation for underlying medical conditions (see page 202). Reassure families that using the police and emergency medical services (eg, calling 911) is the safest and most medically appropriate way of managing violence that places the patient or someone else at risk.

Once an acute episode of violence is under control, or gradually evolving tendencies toward aggression have been evaluated, different strategies can be implemented for long-term management. Divalproex sodium (Depakote®) beginning at doses of 125 mg b.i.d.-t.i.d., and increasing to a total of 1,500 mg or more daily, is recommended.[9] Divalproex sodium is especially useful when psychosis is not a driving factor in the aggression. For milder situations, perhaps after exacerbating factors are ameliorated, trazodone and SSRIs are useful for chronic administration. Some physicians now use other antiepileptic drugs, such as carbamazepine, lamotrigine, and gabapentin, but these are second-line agents usually best reserved for neuropsychiatrists or other dementia specialists familiar with them. For patients with psychotic features as a more important contributor to aggressive acts, consider risperidone, olanzapine, or quetiapine. Cost or other factors may dictate the use of conventional agents, such as haloperidol, but they are generally more toxic at effective antiagitation doses in the dementia population.

Sundowning

Sundowning is a syndrome of restlessness associated with confusion and disorientation. The name sundowning evolved because the behaviors typically begin in the late afternoon or early evening and gradually escalate through the evening hours. Patients wander or exhibit other aberrant motor behaviors, such as pacing or rummaging through drawers. There may also be delusional components known as reduplication, when patients believe that their home is not the 'real' home, or that the caregiver is an impostor who resembles the real caregiver. Fatigue, sensory deprivation (eg, dim light), and disrupted circadian rhythms may all contribute to its evolution.[9] Sundowning is most common in the moderate and severe stages of AD, but can begin earlier. The first-line approach is nonpharmacologic and should include improved sleep hygiene, augmented lighting, and better communication techniques. If these prove inadequate, then trazodone is suggested as the first choice for both short- and long-term management.[9] Divalproex sodium may work if trazodone is ineffective or not well tolerated. Other alternatives include risperidone, olanzapine, or quetiapine, especially when reduplicative phenomena are prominent.

Sleep Disturbance

Sleep disturbance is a common source of distress among dementia caregivers. Increasing patient comfort and limiting the negative effects of disrupted sleep on both patients and caregivers are the goals of drug treatment.[14] Pharmacologic therapy is recommended only when the approaches to sleep hygiene discussed above are unsuccessful. In addition, families should not give over-the-counter sleep agents to the patient. Most agents contain diphenhydramine, a potent antihistaminic, anticholinergic agent. Many AD patients experience paradoxical agitation in response to this class of sedative. Peripheral side effects of anticholinergic activity, such as dry mouth and urinary retention, can add discomfort, further magnifying agitated behavior. Finally, the central nervous system anticholinergic activity magnifies the principal neurochemical deficit associated with AD, which can further worsen cognitive abilities.

Melatonin is another over-the-counter agent marketed as a sleep aid. Many families choose it because it is a natural product. While it may help regulate sleep cycles, it is generally not an acute sedative-hypnotic. Its efficacy in Alzheimer's disease has not been established. Herbal or other natural products have no well-established efficacy in AD and are unlikely to offer any advantage to appropriate nonpharmacologic interventions. In addition, herbal and other 'alternative medicine' products can have unknown adverse effects and drug interactions that complicate their use but are not identified in their labeling or marketing material.

When drug therapy is necessary, consider concomitant symptoms. Poor sleep onset associated with psychotic features, such as paranoid fearfulness, may respond best to an antipsychotic with sedating properties, such as olanzapine. Similarly, depressive rumination preventing sleep is suited to treatment with a sedating antidepressant, like trazodone. When no clear behavioral features complicate the poor sleep, trazodone is recommended as a first choice for both long- and short-term applications.[9] Some clinicians prefer zolpidem (Ambien®) at a bedtime dose of 5 mg to 10 mg.[14] Although it can be hard to find in pharmacies, chloral hydrate—starting at 250 mg at bedtime—is a pure soporific that can help in short-term applications, such as resetting a sleep-wake cycle that has slipped out of phase. Its efficacy fades within weeks and it can lead to gastrointestinal discomfort. Chronic benzodiazepine use for insomnia is not advised.[14]

Conclusions

Behavioral disturbances in dementia present challenges to the clinician. Successful behavioral symptom management entails good listening and communication skills, in order to lead families in the proper administration of both nonpharmacologic and pharmacologic methods. It demands a detailed knowledge of the mechanism and metabolism of the prescribed agents. Successful interventions integrate a curious blend of patience and aggressiveness, a willingness to admit failure, and the determination to try again with a different strategy. When done well, management of behavioral symptoms is genuinely rewarding. In brief, this part of dementia care provides a forum for the true art of medical practice.

References

1.   Geldmacher DS: Delirium, agitation, and confusion. In: Selman WR, Benzel EC, eds. *Neurosurgical Care of the Elderly*. Park Ridge, IL, American Association of Neurological Surgeons, 1999, pp 197-210.

2.   Chan D, Brennan NJ: Delirium: making the diagnosis, improving the prognosis. *Geriatrics* 1999;54:28-30,36,39-42.

3.   Gerber JG, Hollister AS: Drug use in the elderly. In: Jahnigen DW, Schier RW, eds. *Geriatric Medicine*, 2nd ed. Cambridge, MA, Blackwell Science, 1996, pp 84-97.

4.   Klotz U, Avant G, Hoyumpa A, et al: The effects of age and liver disease on the disposition and elimination of diazepam in adult man. *J Clin Invest* 1975;55:347-359.

5.   Sunderland T, Weingartner H, Cohen RM, et al: Low-dose oral lorazepam administration in Alzheimer subjects and age-matched controls. *Pyschopharmacology* 1989;99:129-133.

6.   Grad R: Benzodiazepines for insomnia in community-dwelling elderly: a review of benefit and risk. *J Fam Pract* 1995;41: 473-481.

7.   Satlin A: Sleep disorders in dementia. *Psychiatric Ann* 1994; 24:186-191.

8.   Wimo A, Mattsson B, Adolfsson R, et al: Dementia day care and its effects on symptoms and institutionalization—a controlled Swedish study. *Scand J Prim Health Care* 1993;11:117-123.

9.   Alexopoulos GS, Silver JM, Kahn DA, et al, eds: *The Expert Consensus Guideline series: Treatment of Agitation in Dementia. A Postgraduate Medicine Special Report*. Minneapolis, MN, McGraw-Hill, 1998.

10.   Doody RS, Stevens JC, Beck C, et al: Practice parameter: management of dementia (an evidence-based review). Report of

the Quality Standards Subcommittee of the American Academy of Neurology. *Neurology* 2001;56(9):1154-1166.

11. Ripich DN: Functional communication with AD patients: a caregiver training program. *Alzheimer Dis Assoc Disord* 1994;8: 95-109.

12. Ancoli-Israel S, Klauber MR, Gillin JC, et al: Sleep in non-institutionalized Alzheimer's disease patients. *Aging* 1994;6: 451-458.

13. Miles LE, Dement W: Sleep and aging. *Sleep* 1980;3:1-220.

14. Practice guideline for treatment of patients with Alzheimer's disease and other dementias of late life. American Psychiatric Association. *Am J Psychiatry* 1997;154:1-39.

15. White H, Pieper C, Schmader K: The association of weight change in Alzheimer's disease with severity of disease and mortality: a longitudinal analysis. *J Am Geriatr Soc* 1998;46:1223-1227.

16. Finley B: Nutritional needs of the person with Alzheimer's disease: practical approaches to quality care. *J Am Diet Assoc* 1997; 97:S177-S180.

17. Reifler BV, Teri L, Raskind M, et al: Double-blind trial of imipramine in Alzheimer's disease patients with and without depression. *Am J Psychiatry* 1989;146:45-49.

18. Scharre DW, Chang SI: Cognitive and behavioral effects of quetiapine in Alzheimer disease patients. *Alzheimer Dis Assoc Disord* 2002;16(2):128-130.

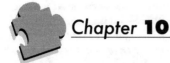

Chapter 10

Interdisciplinary Management of AD

by Elizabeth A. Crooks, RN, MSN, CCRN, CS
Stephen J. Modafferi, JD
and David S. Geldmacher, MD

Patients with dementia have extensive needs, but the pharmacologic management of the illness is limited. The clinical syndrome of Alzheimer's disease is treatable, but its management is complex and extends beyond the traditional bounds of medical practice. While medicine has historically focused on effects of the disease on the patient, dementia treatment requires a broader focus that includes the effect of symptoms on patients and caregivers. This means that physicians must consider the quality of life of both patients and caregivers more than in most diseases. Many of the most effective interventions are nonpharmacologic and can be provided by professionals from many disciplines. Families coping with dementing illness often seek services from several healthcare providers and social service agencies, as well as lawyers and financial planners. The primary care physician must often direct the family to these services. Drawing on resources in the community can dramatically reduce the burden of care for both the family and doctor.

The ideal approach to care of the AD patient is both multidisciplinary and interdisciplinary. Multidisciplinary care refers to parallel services with little direct interaction between providers. A person who sees a doctor, attends a support group, and gets legal advice from an attorney with little or no interaction between these providers receives multidisciplinary care. Interdisciplinary care involves collaboration between care providers who form a team. Ideally, this team is composed of a physician, nurse, social worker, and other allied health specialists as needed. Because interdisciplinary teams cooperate in ways that can blur distinctions between traditional disciplines, leadership of such a team is enhanced when the members understand each other's contributions and areas of expertise.

This chapter gives primary care providers information to trigger an interdisciplinary approach to care of dementia patients. It focuses on the patient and caregiver experience of living with Alzheimer's disease. Strategies to identify problems amenable to interdisciplinary intervention are outlined and team member responsibilities are described. Referral suggestions are made for common problems associated with dementing illness.

The Caregiver Experience

Clinicians must consider families and communities when treating patients with dementia. While it is customary for medical care to focus on the patient, the focus of interdisciplinary care is on the quality of life for the patient within their family unit and community. The interdisciplinary team's objective is to optimize the patient's ability to function and support the caregiver and other family members in their efforts to maintain a safe and satisfying environment. It is important, therefore, to understand the caregiver experience to appreciate the complexities of interdisciplinary management.

About 80% of long-term care for patients with Alzheimer's disease is provided by informal (ie, unpaid) caregivers.[1] These caregivers are usually family members. They have been called the 'hidden victims' because they shoulder the burden of managing the physical, social, and emotional problems that result from Alzheimer's

Table 1: MBRC Caregiver Strain Instrument

The following items refer to how a caregiver feels and behaves as a result of providing care. Please use the following scale to answer questions 1 to 14. There are no right or wrong answers.

- Strongly agree = 3
- Agree = 2
- Disagree = 1
- Strongly disagree = 0

During the past 4 weeks, because of helping the patient, I felt:

1. ___ unsure whether he/she was getting proper care.
2. ___ uncertain about how to best care for him/her.
3. ___ that I should be doing more for him/her.
4. ___ that I could do a better job of caring for him/her.
5. ___ that he/she tried to manipulate me.
6. ___ that my relationship with him/her was strained.
7. ___ that he/she made requests over and above what he/she needed.
8. ___ resentful toward him/her.
9. ___ angry toward him/her.
10. ___ that my physical health was worse than before.
11. ___ downhearted, blue, or sad more often.
12. ___ more nervous or bothered by nerves than before.
13. ___ I had less 'pep' or energy.
14. ___ bothered more by aches and pains.

disease.[2] The traditional responsibility of giving care has fallen to women; only 27% of caregivers are men.[3] Most often, it is the spouse who assumes the role of caregiver,

Caregiver Mastery Score _____ (sum of items 1-4)
Relationship Strain Score _____ (sum of items 5-9)
Health Strain Score _____ (sum of items 10-14)

Please use the following scale to answer questions 15 to 19. There are no right or wrong answers.

- Less often = 2
- The same = 1
- Strongly disagree = 0

During the past four weeks, because of helping the patient, I:
15. ___ participated in church or religious activities.
16. ___ visited with friends or family.
17. ___ participated in group or organized activities.
18. ___ engaged in volunteer activities.
19. ___ went out to dinner, the theater, or a show.

Activity Restriction Score _____ (sum of items 15-19)

No exact cutting points for heightened caregiver risk have been determined for this tool. Answers can help caregivers describe difficulties they are experiencing and, with repeated administrations, can be used to assess change in the care situation over time. However, scores greater than 8 for mastery, greater than 10 for relationship strain or health strain, or greater than 5 for activity restriction may indicate heightened risk and may warrant further clinical investigation.

Source: Margaret Blenkner Research Center, Benjamin Rose Institute, Cleveland, Ohio

although it is not uncommon for it to be the patient's adult child. Regardless of relationship to the patient, caregiving alters family dynamics and requires family members to take on roles for which they may be ill-prepared. As family dynamics change, longstanding conflicts can be exacerbated. To assist the family as they adapt to caregiving, it is necessary to assess their social and emotional resources, as well as their coping styles.

Caregiving Approach

Gender differences affect caregivers. North American men and women are socialized differently to caregiving roles. Women are traditionally socialized to assume caregiving duties and to receive minimal assistance from men.[4] Women caregivers, especially those older than 65 who hold the traditional view that a woman's role is in the home, have difficulty balancing work and family responsibilities.[5] These women handle stressful duties as a labor of love while sacrificing their own needs. They often suppress feelings of anger, pain, and resentment and feel intense guilt when they acknowledge these emotions. This attitude makes it difficult to uncover caregiver problems during an interview. One strategy to overcome this is giving the caregiver 'permission' to express her frustrations in managing the patient. Alternatively, the caregiver can complete the Margaret Blenkner Research Center (MBRC) Caregiver Strain Instrument[6] while in the waiting area or while the patient is examined. This tool (Table 1) is brief and can be given repeatedly to monitor a caregiver's ability to cope. It also provides clues for referrals.

Unlike women, who usually assume all caregiving responsibilities, male caregivers are more likely to delegate duties and use outside services for both household and patient management. They usually have a task-oriented approach that allows a balance of work, rest, and leisure.[4] Although the approach to caregiving differs greatly between men and women, all caregivers experience emotional and physical strain. Research indicates that caregiver style and response to the caregiver role is influenced not only by gender, but also by age, ethnicity, and relationship to the patient.

Depression and Caregiver Health

Clinical depression is reported in about half of primary caregivers, with women at the greatest risk.[7] At the same time, women are less likely to seek help in coping with caregiver burden.

Several factors contribute to the development of clinical depression in caregivers. Their sleep patterns are often disrupted when patients develop day/night reversal. Caregivers must cope with the patient's agitation, unpredictable and disruptive behavior, paranoid ideation, and wandering. As the dementing illness progresses, caregivers must assume physical burdens such as patient bathing, feeding, and toileting. Caregivers commonly suffer fatigue, diminished appetite, and weight loss. Not surprisingly, caregiver depression increases with the patient's dementia severity.[7] Caregivers also report feeling helpless, like they are losing control, anger, stress, and social isolation.[8] Somatic symptoms, such as headache and gastrointestinal problems, have been reported. Caregiver burden can also lead to increased morbidity, which includes ulcers, hypertension, myocardial infarction, and immune compromise.[9]

Managing Caregiver Strain

Predicting caregiver burden is problematic. A linear relationship between caregiver burden and patient impairment is not supported in the literature.[10] Caregiver burden is multifactorial and linked to variables such as availability of social support and financial resources, coping abilities, and feelings of self-efficacy.[11] Considering the devastating emotional and physical costs of caregiving, it is important to create a plan that helps the caregiver recognize his or her limitations, set boundaries for self-sacrifice, and establish a caregiving approach that includes a predictable daily routine. Ideally, this routine conserves physical and emotional resources and makes use of outside sources of support. To do this, the health-care provider must have a clear understanding of the problems challenging the patient and caregiver.

Table 2: Functional Activities Questionnaire (FAQ)

The FAQ is an informant-based measure of functional abilities.[12] Informants provide performance ratings of the target person on 10 complex higher-order activities.

Individual Items of the FAQ

1. ___ Writing checks, paying bills, balancing checkbook
2. ___ Assembling tax records, business affairs, or papers
3. ___ Shopping alone for clothes, household necessities, or groceries
4. ___ Playing a game of skill, working on a hobby
5. ___ Heating water, making a cup of coffee, turning off stove
6. ___ Preparing a balanced meal
7. ___ Keeping track of current events
8. ___ Paying attention to, understanding, and discussing a TV show, book, or magazine
9. ___ Remembering appointments, family occasions, holidays, and medications
10. ___ Traveling out of neighborhood, driving, or arranging to take buses

Total _____

Problem Identification

In assessing patient problems, the clinician should focus on physical, emotional, and social difficulties, as well as those that can arise as the illness advances. Considering potential problems provides a framework for planning patient care and enables the health professional, patient, and caregiver to approach treatment proactively rather than reactively. Anticipating problems also allows for early referral and more effective patient manage-

The levels of performance assigned range from dependence to independence and are rated as follows:

• Dependent = 3

• Requires assistance = 2

• Has difficulty but does by self = 1

• Normal = 0

Two other response options can also be scored.
• Never did (the activity), but could do now = 0
• Never did, and would have difficulty now = 1

A total score for the FAQ is computed by simply summing the scores across the 10 items. Scores range from 0 to 30. A cutpoint of 9 (dependent in 3 or more activities) is recommended.

Pfeffer et al: *J Gerontol* 1982;37:323-329. Copyright © The Gerontological Society of America. Modified by permission of the publisher.[12]

ment. AD caregivers highly value this kind of anticipatory guidance.

One of the hallmarks of dementia is patients' lack of awareness about their own self-care. As the dementing illnesses progress, patients become less able to maintain their family and community roles. At the same time, they are unaware of the extent of their disability. It is important, then, that management of the patient with dementia occurs in cooperation with family or caregivers. Since caregivers frequently identify medical, emotional, and social issues that require intervention, they must be included when clinicians develop an interdisciplinary plan of care.

Functional Ability

Screening for medical problems is done during the history and physical examination. Since the screening primarily focuses on the patient's physical presentation, emotional and social issues affecting patients and caregivers can be overlooked. Clinicians can screen for problems amenable to interdisciplinary intervention with use-structured screening tools and a caregiver/family interview. Initial assessment of functional impairment is done with the Functional Activities Questionnaire (FAQ),[12] which is recommended by the US Clinical Practice Guideline for early identification of dementia.[13] The FAQ (Table 2) is a brief survey that evaluates a patient's performance on 10 complex activities of daily living. Since the patient may be unable to accurately describe his or her abilities, the questionnaire should be given when a family member or other caregiver is present.

An FAQ score of 9 or more, showing dependency in 3 or more activities, is an indication of functional impairment that requires further evaluation. Administering this questionnaire and follow-up interview need not require physician time, because another member of the health-care team or the caregiver can complete it. Although the FAQ is not diagnostic of Alzheimer's disease, it does provide the health-care provider with valuable clues about the types of services the patient or caregiver needs. For instance, difficulties in managing business or financial affairs may indicate a legal referral. Problems with meal preparation may require an occupational therapist, nutritionist, or custodial nursing referral. Along with the FAQ, the Index of Activities of Daily Living[14] (Table 3) provides information about the patient's ability to manage basic and burdensome self-care activities, as well as the type of assistance the caregiver needs.

Table 3: Index for Activities of Daily Living[14]

Please circle the response that you feel best represents the patient's ability to do each of the following activities of daily living.

Activity	Needs no assistance or supervision	Needs some assistance or supervision	Totally dependent/ cannot do at all
Eating	0	1	2
Toileting	0	1	2
Bathing (sponge, shower, or tub)	0	1	2
Dressing	0	1	2
Grooming (combing, shampooing hair; shaving; trimming nails)	0	1	2
Ambulating/ transferring	0	1	2
Total Score			

Other Needs and Family Resources

A member of the interdisciplinary team should ask other important questions about resources and needs early in the course of care (Table 4). This information is used to supplement the information obtained in the FAQ and

Table 4: Other Questions to Determine Caregiver Needs and Resources

1. Do you have a family attorney?
2. Do you have a living will that identifies a health-care proxy?
3. Is your estate planning complete?
4. Do you have legal claims pending?
5. Have you recently entered into a contract that has not been reviewed by your attorney?
6. Have your insurance policies been reviewed recently?
7. Is your will up-to-date?
8. Do you plan to use in-home caregivers?
9. Are you a member of a formal religious organization?
10. What is the source of your spiritual strength or meaning?
11. How do you practice your spiritual beliefs?
12. Has the patient's illness affected your spiritual beliefs?
13. Do you have a spiritual leader?
14. Are you able to maintain your usual religious activities?
15. Do you find your religious group supportive?
16. Are you comfortable contacting your spiritual leader for assistance in managing the demands of caregiving?

Index of ADL. These questions primarily target the legal and spiritual well-being of patients or caregivers. Health-care providers should carefully review responses on the assessment tools, because they form the database upon which referrals are made. Confirmation of the responses should be made during the patient/caregiver interviews and by direct observation of the patient. Along with developing an understanding of patient and caregiver deficits, health-care professionals must explore the meaning of these deficits to the individual and his or her emotional reaction to them.[15] A clear understanding of what the patient and his or her family are thinking and feeling allows the health-care professional to mobilize the interdisciplinary team and address the identified problems.

Interdisciplinary Team Construction, Leadership, and Member Contributions

Interdisciplinary teams can have a formal structure with clearly defined membership and appointed leadership or, as is often the case, an informal structure that differs by patient need and member responsibilities. Time, financial, and human resources, as well as organizational commitment, dictate team construction. Regardless of structure, successful teams are characterized by a shared commitment to quality care and an appreciation for the contributions of each member.[16]

Team coordination can be time-consuming and requires organization, strong communication skills, and the ability to manage conflict. While team leadership can fall to any member, a registered nurse or social worker as team leader frees the physician to focus on medical management. Interdisciplinary case management services may be available in the community through hospital-based social work or home-care departments, independent home health-care agencies (eg, Visiting Nurses), charitable organizations (eg, Catholic Charities, Jewish Family Services), and proprietary case management companies. In addition, local chapters of the Alzheimer's Association can help coordinate dementia-related services.

Table 5: NCCC and Alzheimer's Association Guidelines for Medical Care of Dementia Patients

	Initial identification phase
Goal formation	• Establish treatment goals to optimize health and function for the patient in conjuction with patient/caregiver • Specify time frames for reaching goals
Interventions	Consider: • Additional diagnostic testing • Specialty referrals • Medication changes • Education materials • Audiology referral • Home nursing referral • PT/OT/SLP referrals
Response	• Assess goal attainment • Adjust goals or strategies if goals not met

Source: National Chronic Care Consortium and the Alzheimer's Association.

The Physician's Role

The physician's primary responsibility is diagnosis and medical management of the demented person. This includes a diagnosis of the condition, determination of prognosis,

Longitudinal monitoring and treatment phase	**End-of-life phase**
• Review previous goals and establish new goals in conjunction with patient/caregiver • Specify time frames for reaching goals	• Establish treatment goals to achieve greatest patient/caregiver satisfaction regarding symptom management • Specify time frames for reaching goals
Consider: • Previous interventions	Consider: • Previous interventions • Hospice referral • Chaplaincy referral • Social work referral
• Assess goal attainment • Adjust goals or strategies if goals not met	• Assess goal attainment • Adjust goals or strategies if goals not met

(continued on next page)

and the use of medicines to treat the disease and underlying symptoms. The physician is also frequently responsible for providing the family and patient with referrals for management of problems that cannot be addressed by medication.

Table 5: NCCC and Alzheimer's Association Guidelines for Medical Care of Dementia Patients (continued)

	Initial identification phase
Pathway outcome	Patient receives optimal medical care consistent with accepted standards of care and patient/caregiver preferences
Assessment	• Perform (review) dementia and general assessment (see second component) • Record assessment results in chart including medical problem list, medications, pertinent physical exam, MMSE, vision/hearing screen, laboratory results • Prioritize symptoms in conjunction with patient/caregiver

Longitudinal monitoring and treatment phase

Patient receives optimal medical management with emphasis on secondary and tertiary prevention consistent with accepted standards of care and patient/caregiver wishes

• Evaluate status of previous symptoms
• Assess for new symptoms since last visit
• Review medications for effectiveness, compliance, and potential side effects
• Repeat MMSE every 6 months or sooner as appropriate, until patient scores 10 or less
• Perform focused physical exam based on symptoms/concerns
• Update medical problem list

End-of-life phase

Patient/caregiver satisfied with medical management of symptoms

• Evaluate status of all symptoms
• Review medications for effectiveness, compliance, and potential side effects
• Perform focused physical exam based on symptoms/concerns

Referral from a primary care provider to a subspecialist is not required for all AD cases. Reasons for making referrals to different types of specialists are reviewed in Chapter 6. The National Chronic Care Consortium (NCCC), in cooperation with the Alzheimer's Association, has developed guidelines for the medical management of patients suffering from dementia (Table 5). These guidelines account for progression of the disease by dividing the care into 3 sequential epochs: 1) initial identification, 2) longitudinal monitoring and treatment, and 3) end-of-life.[6]

The Nurse's Role

The nurse's role in caring for demented persons and their caregivers varies based on licensure and scope of practice. The registered nurse (RN) is primarily responsible for the assessment and management of patients' and caregivers' responses to the dementing illness. This includes monitoring symptoms and patient response to medication, meeting the education needs of patients and their caregivers, and assisting them in preparing for disease progression. Professional nursing is based on a conceptual framework that treats the patient in the context of family and community. This philosophical orientation fits well in managing dementia patients. In many institutions, the RN acts as a case manager or interdisciplinary team leader and makes referrals for medical, emotional, and social problems associated with the illness. Along with social workers, registered nurses are skilled at managing patients' and caregivers' psychosocial needs. The NCCC and the Alzheimer's Association guidelines for meeting the psychosocial needs of the patient with dementia are presented in Table 6. Registered nurses and social workers are ideally qualified to implement these guidelines.

Nurse Practitioners (NPs) and Clinical Nurse Specialists (CNSs) are registered nurses with a master's degree or higher, whose scope of practice includes disease diagnosis and prescriptions. They also have a formal education in research and may be involved in clinical trials and other scientific inquiry. These advanced practice nurses may be in solo private practice or a group practice that includes physician partners. The scope of practice for these nurses varies, and is defined by each state's board of nursing. NPs and CNSs often provide a cost-effective approach to management of patients with chronic illness.

A licensed practical nurse (LPN) is trained to provide custodial care, carry out treatments, and administer oral and intravenous medications. These nurses have completed a postsecondary training program and are licensed by each state's board of nursing. The LPN may collect patient data, such as physical presentation and vital signs, but is not qualified to evaluate it. This means the LPN must work under the direct supervision of a physician or registered nurse. The LPN is, however, a good choice for providing in-home custodial care for patients with skilled nursing needs.

Nursing care technicians, who are unlicensed, focus on custodial care. Their responsibilities vary based on their work setting. Nursing care technicians in long-term care settings not only provide custodial care but may also collect patient data, such as vital signs and glucometer readings. In some facilities, they may handle simple procedures such as uncomplicated dressing changes. In acute care settings, they often perform more complex procedures such as urinary catheterization and venipuncture. In the home, these assistants focus on direct patient care and may handle simple housekeeping tasks such as meal preparation.

The Social Worker's Role

Patients with dementing illnesses and their caregivers need access to social services such as respite care, financial services, counseling, and crisis management. Social workers base their practice on the idea that the individual is part of a greater system, and they are prepared to assist the patient and family in acquiring resources needed to cope with the burden of chronic illness.[17] Social workers are also skilled in meeting the emotional needs of people in crisis or facing lifestyle changes.

Table 6: NCCC and Alzheimer's Association Guidelines for Psychosocial Management

	Initial identification phase
Pathway outcome	Patient/caregiver understand monitoring parameters to assess mood and behavioral concerns
Assessment	• Assess patient/caregiver concerns regarding mood, depression, sleep patterns, disruptive behaviors, agitation, aggression, wandering, etc • Administer Geriatric Depression Scale (GDS) • Assess patient/caregiver priorities regarding quality of life issues • Evaluate environmental factors affecting moods/behaviors • Evaluate relationship of activities/schedule to moods/behaviors

Longitudinal monitoring and treatment phase

Patient received optimal management of depression and disruptive behaviors consistent with patient/caregiver wishes

• Evaluate current status of previously identified moods and behavioral problems
• Review available behavior logs/diaries/reports for response to interventions and for new problems
• Reassess for signs of depression
• Update relationship to environment, activity, and other symptoms to moods/behaviors
• Reassess patient/caregiver priorities regarding quality-of-life issues

End-of-life phase

Patient/caregiver satisfied with management strategies used to address moods/behaviors and adjustment to end-of-life

• Assess patient/caregiver satisfaction regarding management of moods/behaviors
• Update previous assessment

(continued on next page)

Table 6: NCCC and Alzheimer's Association Guidelines for Psychosocial Management *(continued)*

	Initial identification phase
Assessment *(continued)*	• Evaluate relationship of other symptoms to moods/behaviors
Goal formation	• Establish methods/ parameters to monitor moods/behaviors • Establish treatment goals for targeted moods/behaviors
Interventions	Consider: • Diary/behavior log • Social work referral • Psychology referral • Support group • Respite care • Home aide • Medications • Family meeting • Educational materials • Chaplaincy materials
Response	• Assess goal attainment • Adjust goals/strategies if goals not met

Source: National Chronic Care Consortium and the Alzheimer's Association.

Longitudinal monitoring and treatment phase	End-of-life phase
• Select management strategies to improve targeted symptoms and moods/behaviors in conjunction with patient/caregiver	• Select management strategies to maximize end-life comfort regarding moods/behaviors in conjunction with patient/caregiver
Consider: • Previous interventions • Behavior management techniques • Changes in medications • Changes in schedule/activities • Changes in environment	Consider: • Previous interventions • Hospice referral
• Assess goal attainment • Adjust goals/strategies if goals not met	• Assess goal attainment • Adjust goals/strategies if goals not met

The patient and family should be referred to a social worker at the time of diagnosis. In many communities, the Alzheimer's Association is equipped to provide this service or identify appropriate referrals to the family. Social workers guide the patient and family through the bureaucracy of health-care reimbursement, identify community agencies available to meet the patient's medical, custodial or skilled nursing, and social needs, and assist them in meeting the emotional challenges of dealing with the presence of a chronic, debilitating, and socially isolating disease.

Illness in a family member alters family dynamics and can create conflicts, but the diagnosis of dementia and the behavioral manifestations of the disease can also exacerbate unresolved emotional issues. Hostility can emerge as the patient becomes more dependent and function declines.[11] The risk for elder abuse increases with the presence of dementia.[18] Although all health-care professionals must be sensitive to the signs of elder abuse, social workers' focus on family relationships and dynamics puts them in a good position to detect it.

Social workers are qualified to provide counseling and support to families as they adapt to role changes, dependency, and conflict. They also have the ability to recognize overt psychopathology and can collaborate with physicians and mental health agencies to get psychiatric care for patients or caregivers. As the dementing illness progresses, social workers explore alternative or long-term placement options with the patient and family. They can also collaborate with clergy and patients' attorneys as they assist the family with end-of-life decisions.[17]

The Physical Therapist's Role

Progressive dementing illnesses frequently cause immobility and complications from lack of activity. These include decreased physical conditioning, loss of muscle strength and tone, poor coordination, and impaired ambulation. The goal of physical therapy is to optimize the patient's physical condition and to maintain ambulation as long as possible. This is a key factor in keeping a patient at home and delaying institutionalization.

Physical therapy may be provided at the patient's home or in a clinic. The physical therapist prescribes an exercise and activity program for the patient and educates the caregiver about the plan. The physical therapist also evaluates the need for assistive devices and instructs the patient and caregiver in their use. Physical therapy success depends on the patient's ability to learn and/or comply with the activity plan. In moderate-to-advanced stages of illness, the benefit of physical therapy may be limited because the patient's ability to follow instructions is impaired.[19]

The Occupational Therapist's Role

Occupational therapy plays an important role in aiding the patient and caregiver to adapt to the patient's diminishing ability to manage daily living. An occupational therapist can recommend and demonstrate the use of devices that assist with toileting, eating, dressing, and home management. The goal of occupational therapy is to maintain the patient's independence while easing the caregiver's burden. Adapting to impaired cognitive and physical function also allows the patient to stay at home longer.

Evaluation of driving competency is another crucial contribution of occupational therapy. Driving is an emotionally charged issue for most patients. Many people resist losing this privilege because it represents independence. Referral to a driving evaluation program provides the patient and family with an unbiased assessment of the patient's abilities and protects not only the patient but the community. Many rehabilitation hospitals offer formal driving evaluation programs. These are preferable to state drivers' licensure tests or commercial 'driving school' assessments, because the occupational therapist/driving evaluator is able to view the patient's performance from a more sophisticated health-care perspective, as well as understand the likely prognosis for any areas of concern in driving ability.

Table 7: NCCC and the Alzheimer's Association Guidelines for Patient Nutrition

	Initial identification phase
Pathway outcome	Patient in ideal body weight range
Assessment	• Evaluate patient/ caregiver status and wishes re: nutritional status • Evaluate diet and nutritional status • Assess eating function • Evaluate how food is obtained and prepared • Obtain history of weight changes • Measure weight • Evaluate for edema and hydration • Evaluate dentition • Evaluate pharmaceutical/ nutrient interactions
Goal formation	• Establish weight/nutritional goals in conjunction with patient/caregiver • Establish home monitoring parameters in conjunction with patient/caregiver • Specify time frame for reaching goals

Longitudinal monitoring and treatment phase	End-of-life phase
Patient maintaining targeted body weight	Patient/caregiver satisfied with diet and nutritional status
• Evaluate for change since last assessment	• Adjust goals to maximize patient/caregiver satisfaction
• Adjust weight and nutritional goals as appropriate, in conjunction with patient/caregiver	• Evaluate for changes since last assessment • Reassess advanced directives re: feeding/ nutritional issues with patient/caregiver

(continued on next page)

Table 7: NCCC and the Alzheimer's Association Guidelines for Patient Nutrition
(continued)

	Initial identification phase
Interventions	Consider: • Swallowing evaluation • Dietitian referral • Nutritional supplements • Diet changes • Home-delivered or other meals program • Social work referral • Caregiver education material • Dental referral
Response	• Assess goal attainment • Adjust strategy if goals not met

Source: National Chronic Care Consortium and the Alzheimer's Association; revised April 1999.

The Nutritionist's Role

Dementia patients are at risk for malnutrition and dehydration caused by confusion, distractibility, and memory loss. In later stages of Alzheimer's disease, the patient experiences sensory-motor impairment that results in dysphagia and an inability to eat independently. As the disease progresses, weight loss is expected.[20] Concomitant health problems common to older adults, such as congestive heart failure, renal disease, and diabetes, make dietary management a challenge. Dietary intake is not only a medical issue; it is a quality-of-life issue. Food has emotional and social meaning beyond nutrition. A successful approach to

Longitudinal monitoring and treatment phase	End-of-life phase
Consider:	Consider:
• Previous interventions	• Previous interventions
	• Feeding tube (only if consistent with patient/ caregiver wishes and goals)
	• Hospice referral
• Assess goal attainment	• Assess goal attainment
• Adjust strategy if goals not met	• Adjust strategy if goals not met

maintaining the patient's nutritional level must, therefore, incorporate the patient's and caregivers' food values. The goal is to maintain the patient's ideal body weight and nutritional well-being without compromising quality of life.

Physicians must often relax strict and unpalatable low-fat/low-salt diet orders in patients with AD to maintain a stable body weight and promote quality of life. This approach is justified by several factors, including the potential loss of flavor perception in AD, the inexorable weight loss that characterizes the disease, and the fact that AD, rather than cardiovascular morbidity, is the primary determinant of life expectancy in these individuals.

Registered dietitians (RD) can identify nutritional deficits and create a plan to ensure adequate caloric intake. They are also able to explore the meaning food holds in the patient's and family's lives, and develop a strategy that incorporates food preferences and family ritual. The RD is also a valuable resource when the family makes decisions on continued nutrition at end of life. There are NCCC/Alzheimer's Association guidelines for meeting the nutritional needs of patients with dementia across the phases of care (Table 7).

The Clergy's Role

Everyone has a spiritual dimension from which they assign meaning to their life. About 75% of elderly persons are members of a religious organization, although they may not regularly attend formal services or meetings.[21] Although organized religion provides a framework for understanding the meaning of existence, people who do not consider themselves affiliated with a particular religion may still feel very spiritually fulfilled. The diagnosis of a serious illness, particularly one that is not curable and will result in disability and death, may predispose patients, their caregivers, and other family members to spiritual distress. Spiritual distress is the state in which an individual or group experiences a disturbance in the belief or value system that provides strength, hope, and meaning to life.[22]

Spiritual distress may manifest itself in several ways. Commonly, the person questions the meaning of life, death, suffering, and the credibility of his or her belief system.[22] This questioning may be accompanied by feelings of anger, resentment, and fear. People experiencing spiritual distress may also withdraw from their usual practice of religious rituals and express a sense of spiritual ambivalence or emptiness. The social isolation that occurs with progressive dementia can also make it difficult for patients and their caregivers to sustain fellowship within a religious community.

**Table 8: Suggestions to Improve
           Nutritional Intake**

Suggest that the family simplify mealtime by:

- Avoiding distractions such as television or multiple conversations during meals

- Setting the table plainly and avoiding extra place settings or utensils

- Providing finger foods if utensils are difficult for the patient to use

- Offering small meals 5 or 6 times a day rather than large meals 3 times a day

*Encourage caregivers to help the patient stay
on task by:*

- Providing soft foods that are easy to chew and swallow

- Reporting chewing or swallowing difficulties to the health-care team

- Staying with the patient during meals

- Gently reminding the patient of the next step with simple instructions, such as: "It is time to swallow," or "It is time to take another bite."

*Assess how comorbidities may be contributing to
weight loss, such as:*

- Problems with dentition

- Swallowing disorders

- Malignancy

- Medications that produce anorexia, including:

    -Acetylcholinesterase inhibitors
    -Antidepressants
    -Antiparkinsonian agents

Table 9: Common Legal Considerations of Alzheimer's Patients

- Advance directives with right-to-die provisions
- Analysis of pending legal claims
- Criminal and reference checks on home-care assistants
- Development of revocable living trust
- Estate and tax planning, including guardianship evaluation and application
- Insurance analysis
- Personal property summary and analysis
- Real property summary and analysis
- Review of current will

Since the goal of interdisciplinary care is to enhance quality of life, it is important to consider the spiritual resources available to patients and their caregivers. It is also necessary to consider the role clergy may play when the patient and family address end-of-life decisions. Consulting with clergy helps patients and their caregivers face life-prolonging options in the face of disease advancement. Families must make decisions about care and the treatment of potentially life-threatening illnesses as they arise. They not only witness, but also participate in, the patient's dying.[6] Clergy and lay ministers help the family address these ethical issues within the context of their faith and culture. They are also able to marshal resources within the religious community to support the patient and caregiver.

Clergy are an excellent resource for anticipatory grief management and bereavement care. Patients with dementia and their families face continuous loss throughout the disease. They must cope with the loss of cognitive and physical function, as well as with the loss of relationships and social standing. They must deal with the grief of current losses while anticipating greater losses in the future. Clergy help the family and patient make sense of this experience, assign it meaning, and proceed with grief.

Ideally, the patient and family should be referred for spiritual guidance to the leader of their religious community, with whom they already have a relationship. When this is not possible, the patient and caregiver should be informed of options for pastoral care available from local congregations in their faith tradition, the chaplain or department of pastoral care at their local hospital, the local chapter of the National Council of Churches, or the local chapter of the Alzheimer's Association.

Legal Issues and the Lawyer's Role

Diagnosis of a dementing illness seriously threatens the patient's and family's social and economic well-being. Consulting with an attorney who specializes in elder or family law is strongly recommended at diagnosis. The attorney makes an important contribution to the patient's care by providing guidance in planning for disability. Legal services are focused on safeguarding the patient's and family's assets, protection from abuse and exploitation, and preserving the patient's rights. Legal considerations for patients with Alzheimer's disease are listed in Table 9.

One of the primary legal concerns for a patient with dementing illness is a mechanism that provides for substitute decision-making.[23] This mechanism may take the form of a guardianship, power of attorney, or trust.[24] Designing a legal plan, however, is challenging if the patient has diminished capacity. Capacity is the ability to understand the nature and effects of one's acts and is a fundamental element in the formation of contracts, execution of wills, and commission of criminal acts. The diagnosis of Alzheimer's disease or a similar dementing illness does not mean the person is incapacitated or unable to initiate a particular legal action. It is imperative, then, that the attorney judge whether the Alzheimer's patient has the capacity to retain him or her and whether that judgment is sufficient to meet the goals of representation.[23] As the disease progresses, capacity diminishes and the person's ability to learn and retain new information, handle complex tasks, reason, behave appropriately, and communicate becomes impaired. The attorney should consult with the patient's physician to determine the client's capacity.

Attorneys should also consider the client's ability to articulate reasons behind their decisions, appreciate the consequences of those decisions, and consider the client's state of mind when determining capacity.[23] The attorney must understand the relationships that define the individual, judge whether his or her decisions are consistent with lifetime commitments, and ensure that the client's voice is heard.

The realization that a time will come when the patient will no longer be competent to make his or her own decisions is a painful one for the entire family. Identifying someone who will assume guardianship for the patient's personal and financial decisions can be emotionally difficult. A guardian is a person or institution appointed by the court to manage the personal or financial affairs of another. The probate court determines if the ward is incompetent and sets the terms of guardianships. Guardianships may include broad powers or they may be limited to specific situations, such as providing consent for medical procedures. Some guardianships are limited to management of personal matters while others focus on the estate and financial affairs.[24] The guardian of the person and the estate may be the same person.

Guardianships have several advantages. They can be obtained quickly with little advance planning to safeguard an incompetent person or his or her estate from immediate injury. They allow for the removal of the incompetent person from an unsafe living environment despite his or her objections. The incompetent person's assets are protected from abuse and the court can provide protection and supervision. Guardianships also clearly identify decision makers for health-care, personal, and financial issues. While guardianships have many advantages, they can be expensive and limiting. Court costs, legal and guardian's fees, and bond premiums may be incurred. Estate planning may be limited by the court's refusal to approve asset transfer. To avoid the expense and bureaucracy of guardianships, families often use legal alternatives, such as durable power of attorney or living trust, to manage the patient's personal and financial affairs.

The most common device used to privately manage a patient's legal affairs is the durable power of attorney (DPA). This document authorizes someone to act as the legal agent or 'attorney-in-fact' for the patient and it is 'durable' because it remains effective even after the patient becomes incapacitated. To create a power of attorney, the patient must be competent at the time of signing. This requires advance planning and anticipation of future needs.

Careful consideration must be given to the development of the DPA because it is likely to be used for many years. The patient must consider the ability and trustworthiness of the attorney-in-fact to manage his or her personal and financial affairs and whether the attorney-in-fact can appoint someone else to fulfill those responsibilities. It must also be decided whether the DPA should take effect immediately or whether it should be a 'springing' power of attorney that becomes effective only on incapacity or disability. In a springing DPA, the definition of incapacity and disability must be established. Since a DPA does not provide instructions for asset management, the patient must decide whether the attorney-in-fact should be required to give accountings and whether compensation will be made for the service. Most importantly, the patient must completely trust the person chosen to act as his or her agent. Although the essence of the DPA is to grant powers to the attorney-in-fact, state laws

Table 10: NCCC and Alzheimer's Association Guidelines for Advance Directives Planning

	Initial identification phase
Pathway outcome	Patient/caregiver understand purpose of advance directives/ living will/durable power of attorney for health care
Assessment	• Assess patient/ caregiver readiness to discuss advance directives • Assess patient values/ agenda regarding medical treatment • Assess patient ability to understand advance directives • Evaluate patient/caregiver knowledge regarding advance directives • Assess for conflict or inconsistencies in treatment wishes

may restrict these powers. In addition, some financial institutions, such as banks, insurance companies, and investment programs, may refuse to act upon an attorney-in-fact's directions, or place cumbersome limitations on his or her authority.[23]

Longitudinal monitoring and treatment phase

Patient/caregiver enact advance directive as legally allowed according to cognitive status

• Evaluate patient/caregiver need for additional information
• Review decisions regarding advance directives, statements regarding treatment wishes, limitations, etc with patient/caregiver as appropriate
• Repeat elements of original identification phase assessment for patient/caregiver, if previously deferred or declined

End-of-life phase

Patient/caregiver wishes regarding end-of-life care are followed

• Evaluate for changes in patient/caregiver wishes regarding treatment decisions
• Assess for conflicts among patient/family members/caregivers

(continued on next page)

A DPA gives broad powers to the attorney-in-fact to manage the patient's personal and financial affairs. In comparison, a living trust is a legal document that creates a fund from the patient's assets used to benefit the patient or his or her spouse and children. The patient appoints a trustee

Table 10: NCCC and Alzheimer's Association Guidelines for Advance Directives Planning *(continued)*

	Initial identification phase
Goal formation	Provide information/documents to patient/caregiver according to identified needs
Interventions	Consider: • Education materials • Social work referral • Chaplaincy referral • Psychology referral • Legal counsel • Support group referral
Response	• Verify that information/documents are received and reviewed • Adjust strategy if goal not met

Source: National Chronic Care Consortium and the Alzheimer's Association, revised April 1999.

whose primary duty is to apply the income and assets of the trust to the patient's comfort, care, and support, as well as to manage the trust. Unlike a DPA, the trust must be managed in accordance with specific instructions that limit the risk of abuse or exploitation. A trust can also be used to

Longitudinal monitoring and treatment phase	End-of-life phase
Obtain copies of advance directive statements regarding treatment wishes, limitations, for chart(s)	• Resolve any conflicts among patient/caregiver/ family members • Maximize patient/ caregiver satisfaction with end-of-life treatment decisions
Consider: • Previous interventions	Consider: • Previous interventions • Hospice referral
• Verify that documents are on chart • Adjust strategy if goal not met	• Assess goal attainment • Adjust strategies if goal not met

distribute remaining assets upon the patient's death to avoid the expense and inconvenience of probate court.

The cost of establishing a living trust is generally higher than that of a DPA, but the trustee is usually more accepted by third parties as a decision maker. A trust is designed only to manage assets. This means that the need for a guardian may not be eliminated. Finally, the patient must be competent at the time the trust is executed, which requires advance planning.

Although the most urgent legal considerations for patients with Alzheimer's disease are providing a mechanism that safeguards their rights, gives them a voice in directing their own care, and provides for their comfort and support, other issues should be reviewed with an attorney. These issues include estate planning, asset inventory and plans for transfer upon death, and Medicare planning. Legal claims should be reviewed and the patient and family counseled about the ability of the patient to enter into future contracts. An attorney can also coordinate background investigations of candidates for employment as home health aides and housekeepers.

Advance Directives

One of the most difficult things patients and their families must face is the terminal nature of Alzheimer's disease and the resulting severe physical disability. An advance directive is a document that provides patients with the ability to make decisions on life-sustaining treatments and procedures before they are unable to speak for themselves. Issues the patient and family face when establishing an advance directive are both ethical and legal. The patient must decide whether he or she wants nutrition, hydration, and other life-sustaining treatments withheld or withdrawn. Patients may also designate a person to make health-care decisions for them if they cannot speak for themselves through a durable power of attorney for health-care. To avoid conflicts of interest, this health-care proxy should not be a physician or a member of an institution involved in the patient's care unless he or she is a blood relative. In addition, state laws vary regarding the ability of the health-care proxy to refuse or withdraw consent for life-maintaining procedures. As with DPAs and living trusts, an advance directive requires that the patient be competent at the time of execution. The NCCC and the Alzheimer's Association have developed guidelines to assist the patient and caregiver in establishing advance directives. These are depicted in Table 10.

Referral Suggestions

Effective care of the dementia patient hinges on identifying problems early and selecting appropriate management resources. Although the interdisciplinary team provides a wealth of expertise in managing patient and caregiver problems, abundant community resources also exist. The NCCC and the Alzheimer's Association created a guideline for caregiver support that takes disease progression and changing caregiver needs into consideration (Table 11). Common patient and caregiver problems with suggested referrals are listed in Table 12.

Meeting Patient and Caregiver Information Needs

Effective patient and caregiver education depends on the availability of information, which can be provided through discussion. However, written materials should also be available for easy review and future reference. Information may also be provided through structured programs, such as those offered by the Alzheimer's Association or other outreach groups.

Internet resources for information and support have flourished over the last few years. Unfortunately, the accuracy and quality of this information varies. Patients and caregivers should be careful about what information they accept. They should confirm information with their health-care providers and be skeptical of claims that offer cures, or information received from commercial ventures. Table 13 lists some sources for patient and family education and support.

The Alzheimer's Association

The Alzheimer's Association is a national organization whose mission is to support patients with AD and

Table 11: NCCC and Alzheimer's Association Guidelines for Caregiver Support

	Initial identification phase
Pathway outcome	Caregiver(s) are identified and given information and support in accordance with their needs/wishes
Assessment	• Identify current and potential caregivers • Record contact information in patient chart • Assess caregiver's concerns, agenda, needs, and availability • Assess caregiver's knowledge • Assess caregiver's role with ADLs/IADLs • Assess caregiver's perception of patient's living environment (appropriateness and safety)
Goal formation	• Provide caregiver with information, referrals, and resource materials

Longitudinal monitoring and treatment phase

Caregiver(s) are supported to enable them to maximize their caregiving role(s) while maintaining appropriate balance in their personal lives

- Update caregiver information
- Follow up on status of previous caregiver concerns and needs
- Assess for new issues and burdens
- Assess caregiver's role regarding ADLs/IADLs
- Assess caregiver's perception of patient's living environment (appropriateness and safety)

- Review/revise caregiver roles as appropriate according to changing needs in conjunction with patient/caregiver

End-of-life phase

Caregiver(s) achieve maximum satisfaction with their role(s)

- Assess caregiver comfort/concerns with end-of-life issues
- Assess burden of caregiver tasks and need for respite
- Evaluate caregiver's perception of patient's environment regarding appropriateness for meeting end-of-life needs

Adjust caregiver roles by providing additional support services as needed to achieve maximum caregiver satisfaction

(continued on next page)

Table 11: NCCC and Alzheimer's Association Guidelines for Caregiver Support
(continued)

	Initial identification phase
Goal formation *(continued)*	• Establish caregiver role(s) as appropriate in conjunction with patient/caregiver
Interventions	Refer to Alzheimer's Association and consider: • Education materials • Counseling referral • Social work referral • Support group • Respite services/aide services • Family meeting • Other community referrals • Home nursing referrals • PT/OT/SLP referrals • Chaplaincy referral
Response	• Assess goal attainment • Adjust goals/strategies if goals not met

Source: National Chronic Care Consortium and the Alzheimer's Association.

Longitudinal monitoring and treatment phase	End-of-life phase
• Provide caregiver support to maximize ability to fulfill role with appropriate balance and satisfaction	
Refer to Alzheimer's Association and consider: • Previous interventions • Chaplaincy referral	Refer to Alzheimer's Association and consider: • Previous interventions • Hospice referrals
• Assess goal attainment • Adjust goals/strategies if goals not met	• Assess goal attainment • Adjust goals/strategies if goals not met

Table 12: Suggested Referrals for Common Problems

	Physician	Nurse	Social worker	PT	OT	Speech therapist	Nutritionist	Lawyer	Clergy	Alzheimer's Assoc.	Hospice
Custodial Care Issues:											
ADL impairment	•	•			•						
Ambulation difficulty		•		•							
Inadequate oral intake/weight loss	•	•			•	•	•				•
Incontinence	•	•		•							
Home safety		•			•						
Driving/transportation			•		•						
Behavioral Problems:											
Agitation/violent behavior	•	•	•							•	
Forgetfulness	•	•									
Apathy/depression	•	•	•						•	•	•
Delusions/psychosis	•	•									
Wandering	•	•								•	

274

	1	2	3	4	5	6	7	8	9	10
Sleep disturbances	•									•
Communication problems	•	•					•			•
End-of-Life Decisions:										
Advance directives	•			•						•
Estate planning				•						
Financial planning				•						
Family/Caregiver Issues:										
Altered family roles	•	•	•							•
Patient capacity/guardianship	•		•	•						•
Caregiver strain/depression	•	•	•							•
Respite care	•	•								•
Social support	•	•	•							•
Spiritual crisis	•		•							•
Long-term care placement		•	•	•						•

Table 13: Sources for Patient/Caregiver Information

American Association of Retired Persons
601 E Street, NW
Washington, DC 20049
1-800-424-3410
E-mail: member@aarp.org
Web site: www.aarp.org

Administration on Aging
330 Independence Avenue, SW
Washington, DC 20201
1-800- 677-1116 (Eldercare Locator—to find services
for an older person in his or her locality)
FAX: 1-202-260-1012
E-mail: aoainfo@aoa.gov
Web site: www.aoa.dhhs.gov/elderpage.html

Alzheimer's Association
919 North Michigan Avenue, Suite 1100
Chicago, Illinois 60611-1676
1-800-272-3900 or 1-312-335-8700
Fax: 1-312-335-1110
E-mail: info@alz.org
Web site: www.alz.org

**Alzheimer's Disease Education
and Referral Center**
ADEAR Center, PO Box 8250,
Silver Spring, Maryland 20907-8250
1-800-438-4380, Fax: 1-301-495-3334
E-mail: adear@alzheimers.org
Web site: www.alzheimers.org/adearctr.html

EldercareWeb
E-mail: ksb@elderweb.com
Web site: www.elderweb.com

Emotional Support on the Internet
Web site: www.cix.co.uk/~net-services/care/

Institute for Brain Aging and Dementia
The Alzheimer's Disease Research Center, Washington
University
St. Louis, Missouri 63110
1-314-268-2456
E-mail: adrc-info@www.adrc.wustl.edu
Web site: www.biostat.wustl.edu/alzheimer

National Academy of Elder Law Attorneys, Inc.
1604 North Country Club Road
Tucson, Arizona 85716
1-520-881-4005, Fax: 1-520-325-7925
Web site: www.naela.com

National Aging Information Center
330 Independence Avenue, SW, Room 4656
Washington, DC 20201
1-202-619 7501; Fax: 1-202-401-7620
E-mail: naic@aoa.gov
Web site: www.aoa.dhhs.gov/naic/

The National Association for Home Care
2288 Seventh Street, SE
Washington, DC 20003
1-202-547-7424; Fax: 1-202-547-3540
E-mail: webmaster@nahc.org
Web site: www.nahc.org.

National Family Caregivers Association
10400 Connecticut Avenue, #500
Kensington, MD 20895-3944
1-800-896 3650; Fax: 1-301-942 2302
E-mail: info@nfcacares.org
Web site: www.nfcacares.org

their caregivers by acting as a clearinghouse for information, as well as by sponsoring programs for health-care providers. The association has local chapters that provide programs and publications to educate the public about caregiver and medical issues, as well as providing advocacy for people with dementing illness. Local chapters frequently sponsor support groups for caregivers and help identify community resources available to AD patients and their caregivers.

The How to Cope program is sponsored by local chapters and tries to meet the education and information needs of Alzheimer's caregivers. The program is designed to provide information and support for early-to-middle stage caregivers and includes a medical overview, suggestions for managing behavioral manifestations of AD, strategies for meeting the patient's daily living needs, and planning for the long-term consequences of the disease.[25]

The Alzheimer's Association also sponsors the Safe Return program. This nationwide system is designed to help police and private citizens identify, locate, and return people with impaired memories caused by Alzheimer's disease or a related disorder. Caregivers of patients who are at risk for wandering should register their loved ones with Safe Return. When a person registered in Safe Return is lost, his or her family contacts the program's emergency 800 number. Callers receive guidance on searching the area, contacting the police, and reporting the person missing. If necessary, a 'missing person' notice is created and distributed in areas where the person may have traveled. Safe Return stays in contact if a search begins, and afterward to help prevent future wandering. Someone who finds a lost person can call the national 800 number listed on the person's Safe Return identification item (jewelry, clothing label, or wallet card). Contact information for people registered in the program is stored in a national database, accessible to operators 24 hours a day, 7 days a week.

Local Offices of Aging

Many communities have offices of aging that use federal, state, local, and private money to fund and administer services/programs for older adults and their caregivers. Services vary by community. Patients and caregivers should be encouraged to contact the local office of aging for a list of services designed for people suffering from dementing illness.

Alzheimer's Disease Education and Referral (ADEAR) Center

This service of the US National Institute on Aging (NIA) provides news about the latest research findings on Alzheimer's disease and services for patients and their families. The NIA is part of the federal government's National Institutes of Health located in Bethesda, MD.

Established by the NIA in 1990, the ADEAR Center provides information about Alzheimer's disease, its impact on families and health professionals, and research into possible causes and cures.

The toll-free telephone number (800-438-4380) connects the caller with an information specialist who will help answer questions about Alzheimer's disease, provide information about the latest research and treatment, provide access to publications about AD and related disorders, and suggest resources for further information or assistance.

The American Association for Retired Persons (AARP)

The AARP is the nation's leading organization for people age 50 and older. It serves their needs and interests through information and education, advocacy, and community services. A network of local chapters and experienced volunteers throughout the country provides these resources. The AARP has an extensive listing of services available for elders and their caregivers. Some of these services are specifically for people coping with Alzheimer's disease and related disorders.

The National Family Caregivers Association

The National Family Caregivers Association (NFCA) is a national, charitable organization dedicated to making life better for family caregivers. The NFCA reaches across the life cycle and across the boundaries of differing diagnoses and relationships to address the common needs of family caregivers. Through its services in information and education; support and validation; public awareness, and advocacy, the NFCA strives to minimize the disparity between a caregiver's quality of life and that of mainstream Americans.

Respite Care

As previously mentioned, the demands of caregiving can have catastrophic consequences on both the caregiver and the family. It is important, then, that caregiver respite be emphasized as a priority and addressed at each visit. Respite care need not occur in a formal setting. Often, caregivers need only be reminded to marshal the resources available within the extended family or social circles. Be prepared, however, to encounter resistance to respite. Caregivers frequently feel guilty about their negative feelings about the burdens of caregiving and may have difficulty entrusting the care of the patient to another. It is not unusual for a caregiver to experience a crisis before using respite services.[26]

Respite care can be provided in several ways. In its most intensive form, it involves admission to a nursing home or hospital.[11] More often, it entails the use of adult day-care services or companion and home-care services. Other respite options include assisted living communities and board-and-care homes. Use of respite services may delay long-term care placement and have financial benefits beyond that of momentarily relieving caregiver burden.[27]

Skilled Nursing Facilities

There are few treatment recommendations as emotionally difficult as placing a patient in a long-term nursing facility. This possibility should be addressed early and as part of the family's economic long-range planning. The health-care professional must also be sensitive to patients and caregivers from cultures in which institutionalization is unacceptable.

Long-term residential facilities that offer specialized care for dementia patients are commonplace. These facilities are designed to provide a safe environment for the patient, minimize disruptive behaviors, and engage the resident in planned activities.[28] The caregiving family should be made aware that these services exist. A word of caution, however, is necessary. There are no standards that define specialized long-term dementia care. Any facility may advertise itself as having an Alzheimer's care unit. It is essential that families investigate the quality of care provided by the facility by interviewing the administrators, staff, residents, and their family members. Issues such as resident-to-caregiver ratio, caregiver training, and staff turnover should be addressed. The number of support staff should also be evaluated. The daily activity schedule should be reviewed for appropriateness. The schedule should balance sensory-stimulating and sensory-calming activities.[29] These activities may include recreation programs, such as music and art therapy, body movement, and group projects, like gardening or crafts.

Ombudsman Programs

When patients or their caregivers express dissatisfaction with the care received in a long-term care facility, a referral to an ombudsman may help. The word 'ombudsman' is adopted from Swedish and refers to a person who receives and investigates consumer complaints and attempts to develop a cooperative resolution. Ombudsman programs are federally mandated to handle conflict between long-term care facilities and their residents. Information regarding ombudsman programs should be made available when caregivers are considering nursing home placement. Contact information for local ombudsman's offices can usually be provided by county health departments, the neighborhood office on aging outlets, or the Alzheimer's Association.

Hospice Care

Although used primarily by patients with cancer and other terminal illnesses, hospice care is available in some communities for patients with end-stage dementia. These programs focus on providing comfort for the dementia patient using psychosocial and environmental therapies.[29] Patients in end-stage dementia are unable to participate in group activities, experience physical complications associated with dementia, and may no longer be ambulatory. This makes them poor candidates for care within a specialized Alzheimer's unit. Hospice care should be considered when the patient no longer benefits from the services provided by routine dementia care programs. Hospice philosophy focuses on maintaining the patient's dignity, allows for the natural progression of illness, and promotes engagement and affirmation of life. Support of the family and primary caregiver also is a priority.

Hospice care is available in several settings. It is provided within the home, long-term care facility, or specialized inpatient hospice centers. Assistance in locating a hospice agency within a community can be obtained through the National Association for Home Care (Table 13).

Reference

1.   Pepper Commission: *A Call for Action. U.S. Bipartisan Commission on Comprehensive Health Care.* Washington, DC, US Government Printing Office, 1990.

2.   Eisdorfer C, Rabins PV, Reisberg B: Alzheimer's disease: Caring for the caregiver. *Patient Care* 1991;25:49-59.

3.   National Alliance for Caregiving: *Family Caregiving in the United States: Findings from a National Study.* Bethesda, MD, National Alliance for Caregiving, 1997.

4.   Corcoran MA: Gender differences in dementia management plans of spousal caregivers: implications for occupational therapy. *Am J Occup Ther* 1992;46:1006-1012.

5.   Montgomery RV, Datwyler MM: Women and men in the caregiving role. *Generations* 1990;14:34-38.

6.   National Chronic Care Consortium and the Alzheimer's Association: *Tools for the Assessment and Treatment of Dementia in*

Managed Care Settings. Bloomington MN, National Chronic Care Consortium, 1999.

7.   Gallagher D, Rose J, Rivera P, et al: Prevalence of depression in family caregivers. *Gerontologist* 1989;29:449-456.

8.   Bass DM, McClendon MJ, Deimling GT, et al: The influence of a diagnosed mental impairment on family caregiver strain. *J Gerontol* 1994;49:S146-S155.

9.   Kiecolt-Glaser JK, Glaser R, Shuttleworth EC, et al: Chronic stress and immunity in family caregivers of Alzheimer's disease victims. *Psychosom Med* 1987;49:523-535.

10.   Hadjistavropoulos T, Taylor S, Tuokko H, et al: Neuropsychological deficits, caregivers' perception of deficits and caregiver burden. *J Am Geriatr Soc* 1994;42:308-314.

11.   Dunkin JJ, Anderson-Hanley C: Dementia caregiver burden: A review of the literature and guidelines for assessment and intervention. *Neurology* 1998;51(suppl 1):S53-S60.

12.   Pfeffer R, Kurosaki T, Harrah C Jr, et al: Measurement of functional activities in older adults in the community. *J Gerontol* 1982;37:323-329.

13.   Costa PT Jr, Williams TF, Somerfeld M, et al: *Early Identification of Alzheimer's Disease and Related Dementias. Clinical Practice Guideline, Quick Reference Guide for Clinicians, No. 19.* Rockville, MD, US Department of Health and Human Services, Public Health Service. Agency for Healthcare Policy and Research, AHCPR Publication No. 97-0703, November 1996.

14.   Katz S, Ford AB, Moskowitz RW, et al: Studies of illness in the aged. The index of ADL: a standardized measure of biological and psychosocial function. *JAMA* 1963;185:914-919.

15.   Foley, J: The experience of being demented. In: Binstock RH, Post SG, Whitehouse PJ, eds. *Dementia and Aging: Ethics, Values and Policy Choices.* Baltimore, The Johns Hopkins University Press, 1992.

16.   Verhey FR, Jolles J, Ponds RW, et al: Diagnosing dementia: a comparison between a monodisciplinary and a multidisciplinary approach. *J Neuropsychiatry Clin Neurosci* 1993;5:78-85.

17.   Guttman M, Stober J: The social worker: an important part of the Parkinson multidisciplinary team. *Parkinson Report* 1999: 10; 9-11.

18. Lachs M, Williams C, O'Brien S, et al: Risk factors for reported elder abuse and neglect: a nine-year observational cohort study. *Gerontologist* 1997;37:469-474.

19. Working around dementia. *Mag Phys Ther* 1995;3:64-68, 78-79.

20. Rouse J, Gilster S: An improved method of documenting and evaluating nutritional intake of persons with Alzheimer's disease. *J Nutr Elder* 1994;14:45-55.

21. Matteson AM, McConnell ES: *Gerontological Nursing: Concepts and Practice*. Philadelphia, WB Saunders, 1998.

22. Carpenito LJ: *Nursing Diagnosis: Application to Clinical Practice*, 6th ed. Philadelphia, JB Lippincott Co, 1995.

23. Christopher AM: Initial legal considerations of Alzheimer's patients: Process and form. *Am J Alzheimer's Dis* 1996;11:25-28.

24. Reckman MS, Seiler LH: Mental competency and planning for disability. *Caring* 1991;10:53-56.

25. Steffen AM, Tebb S, McGillick J: How to cope: Documenting the changing information needs of Alzheimer's caregivers. *Am J Alzheimer's Dis* 1999;14:262-269.

26. Lawton M, Brody E, Saperstein A: A controlled study of respite service for caregivers of Alzheimer's patients. *Gerontologist* 1989;29:8-16.

27. Adler G, Ott L, Jelinski M, et al: Institutional respite care: benefits and risks for dementia patients and caregivers. *Int Psychogeriatr* 1993;5;67-77.

28. Swanson EA, Maas ML, Buckwalter KC: Catastrophic reactions and other behaviors of Alzheimer's residents: special units compared with traditional units. *Arch Psychiatr Nurs* 1993;7:292-299.

29. Wilson SA, Kovach CR, Stearns SA: Hospice concepts in the care of end-stage dementia. *Geriatr Nurs* 1996;17:6-10.

Index

Continuing Medical Education Quiz

To apply for CME credits, record your answers on the answer grid of the Registration Form that is attached to the back cover of this book. Follow the instructions at the beginning of this book.

1. The major risk factor for Alzheimer's disease (AD) is:
   a. age
   b. female gender
   c. head injury
   d. amyloid precursor protein (chromosome 21) mutations

2. The apolipoprotein E ε-4 allele represents:
   a. a causative mutation for AD
   b. a risk factor for AD
   c. a protective factor for AD
   d. a recommended part of the assessment of all AD patients

3. The major payer for AD-related costs is:
   a. Medicaid
   b. Medicare
   c. patient and family (ie, out-of-pocket)
   d. private health insurance

4. The senile plaque:
   a. is extracellularly located
   b. is the site of amyloid deposition
   c. includes glial and neuronal components
   d. all of the above

5. Neurofibrillary tangles are:
   a. found only in AD
   b. related to the neuronal cytoskeleton
   c. composed of amyloid-β protein
   d. secreted by microglial cells

6. Which of the following is the most important contributor to cognitive dysfunction in AD?
   a. synaptic loss
   b. neurofibrillary tangles
   c. senile plaques
   d. granulovacuolar degeneration

7. Which of the following most accurately reflects the importance of autosomal-dominant forms of AD?
   a. They represent the most common inheritance pattern.
   b. They are associated with amyloid precursor protein processing.
   c. They are related to APOE genotype.
   d. They are associated with later age of dementia onset.

8. In what percentage of AD patients are specific causative genetic mutations found?
   a. <5%
   b. 10%-20%
   c. 33%-50%
   d. >75%

9. Which of the following most accurately reflects the importance of memory loss dysfunction in AD?
   a. It is sufficient for diagnosing AD.
   b. It is associated with diffuse dysfunction of the cerebral cortex in AD.
   c. It is often the only symptom of AD.
   d. It is the most commonly recognized symptom in AD.

10. Which of the following most accurately reflects the importance of language dysfunction in dementia?
    a. it excludes AD as the cause
    b. it occurs only late in AD's course
    c. it results in empty, clichéd speech
    d. it does not interfere with social relationships

11. Which of the following does *not* make office-based diagnosis of mild AD more difficult?
    a. absence of a family informant in the examination/consultation room
    b. loss of old habits and remote memories
    c. poor insight into impact of deficits on everyday life
    d. preserved social skills and basic personality

12. Which one of the following behavior changes is common in patients with mild AD?
    a. delusions
    b. sundowning
    c. apathy
    d. wandering

13. In making the diagnosis of Alzheimer's disease, practitioners should:
    a. wait for 100% certainty before applying the diagnosis
    b. use published practice parameters and clinical criteria
    c. use cut-off scores on cognitive tests
    d. combine available genotyping and biomarker tests

14. Which statement about nondisabling memory complaints in older adults is most accurate?
    a. They should be dismissed as a normal part of aging.
    b. They are usually caused by TIAs or 'mini-strokes.'
    c. They should be systematically assessed and followed.
    d. They are rarely caused by medications.

15. Which of the following symptoms is most closely associated with dementia with Lewy bodies?
    a. hour-to-hour cognitive fluctuations
    b. early hallucinations
    c. parkinsonism co-emerging with cognitive deficits
    d. all of the above

16. Which of the following symptom patterns is most closely associated with cerebrovascular disease as the cause of dementia?
    a. aphasia, apraxia, agnosia
    b. focal neurologic deficits, urinary dysfunction, gait disorder
    c. gaze paralysis, axial rigidity, falls
    d. neuropathy, myelopathy, psychosis

17. Which one of the following is *not* a recognized cause or aggravator of apparent dementia?
    a. depression
    b. tobacco use
    c. brain tumor
    d. alcohol abuse

18. According to the American Academy of Neurology, which one of the following diagnostic tests should be performed in all patients with suspected AD?
    a. lumbar puncture for spinal fluid analyses
    b. erythrocyte sedimentation rate (ESR)
    c. electroencephalogram (EEG)
    d. thyroid function tests

19. What is the most appropriate action when routine office assessment fails to identify a cause of cognitive impairment in a person with suspected dementia?
    a. obtain urinary biomarker testing
    b. refer to a neuropsychologist
    c. order a brain PET scan
    d. defer decision making until the diagnostic pattern becomes clear

20. Failure to improve cognitive test scores means that a symptomatic dementia therapy is ineffective.
    a. true
    b. false

21. How can therapeutic success in AD therapy be defined?
    a. improvement in cognition
    b. delay in decline
    c. less than expected decline
    d. all of the above

22. Which of the following is *not* generally recognized as a valid domain for assessing response to current dementia therapies?
    a. caregiver report
    b. cerebral volume on CT scan
    c. cognitive test scores
    d. competence in activities of daily living

23. Which one of the following is supported by the literature as effective disease-modifying therapy in AD?
    a. ginkgo biloba
    b. estrogen
    c. vitamin E
    d. nonsteroidal anti-inflammatory drugs (NSAIDs)

24. Among patients with clinically diagnosed mild AD, cholinergic therapy should be delayed for 3-6 months to establish the rate progression on the Mini-Mental State Examination.
    a. true
    b. false

25. Which one of the following is *not* a recognized benefit of cholinesterase inhibitor therapy in patients with AD?
    a. delay long-term care placement
    b. reduce adverse behavior
    c. reduce neuronal death rates
    d. sustain function and cognition

26. In which of the following areas are the approved cholinesterase inhibitors most similar?
    a. efficacy on standard outcomes
    b. adverse effects
    c. pharmacokinetics
    d. reported mechanism of action

27. Based on placebo-controlled and open-label studies, cholinesterase inhibitor therapy offers mean treatment benefits over what time?
    a. <3 months
    b. 3-6 months
    c. 6-12 months
    d. >12 months

28. GI side effects with cholinesterase inhibitor therapy are:
    a. a correlate of acetylcholinergic potency in the brain
    b. a result of the cholinergic action of the cholinesterase agents
    c. cumulative and irreversible
    d. unrelated to dosage

29. Which one of the following should a caregiver *not* do when caring for a person with mild or moderate AD?
    a. reduce complexity in decision-making activities
    b. provide for social interaction outside the home
    c. quiz the patient about recent events to 'exercise' the memory
    d. have the person do household tasks such as folding the laundry

30. What is the most appropriate initial action when an acutely agitated dementia patient is brought to the emergency department?
    a. admit to psychiatry for medication adjustment
    b. call for neurology consultation
    c. check physical examination and laboratory tests for acute medical illness
    d. treat with diazepam 2-5 mg q 1 h until agitation resolves

31. Which one of the following is a possible cause of agitation in patients with AD?
   a. delirium
   b. pain
   c. fatigue
   d. all of the above

32. According to evidence-based and consensus panel recommendations, benzodiazepines are most appropriately used in dementia patients for what type of adverse behavior?
   a. catastrophic behavioral reactions
   b. chronic and recurrent sundowning
   c. episodic anxious symptoms
   d. insomnia and sleep disturbance

33. For the dementia patient with daily agitation related to delusional symptoms unresponsive to redirection, the most appropriate treatment choice would be:
   a. alprazolam 0.5-1.0 mg qhs
   b. diphenhydramine 50 mg q 6 h prn
   c. haloperidol 2-5 mg q 6 h prn
   d. quetiapine 25-50 mg qhs

34. What is the difference between multidisciplinary and interdisciplinary care?
   a. Multidisciplinary care is characterized by parallel services while interdisciplinary care is characterized by collaboration.
   b. Multidisciplinary care is physician directed while interdisciplinary care is nurse directed.
   c. Multidisciplinary care is reimbursable by Medicare while interdisciplinary care is not.
   d. Multidisciplinary care results in better short-term and long-term outcomes than interdisciplinary care.

35. What is the most appropriate way to gauge caregiver strain?
    a. Ask the patient his or her impressions of the caregiver's ability to cope.
    b. Have the office personnel conduct a telephone interview.
    c. Directly observe the caregiver during a patient visit.
    d. Use a standardized evaluation tool confirmed by interview during a patient visit.

36. Which services should be initiated once AD is diagnosed?
    a. nutrition and speech therapy
    b. physical and occupational therapy
    c. social services and legal consultation
    d. clergy and home health nursing

This program is valid until June 30, 2005.

Notes

Notes

Notes

Notes